A PRACTICAL APPROACH TO

MOVEMENT DISORDERS

DIAGNOSIS AND MEDICAL AND SURGICAL MANAGEMENT

· ·

HUBERT H. FERNANDEZ, MD

Associate Professor
Co-Director, Movement Disorders Center
Co-Director, Residency Training Program
Department of Neurology
McKnight Brain Institute
University of Florida College of Medicine
Gainesville, Florida

RAMON L. RODRIGUEZ, MD

Clinical Assistant Professor
Director, Clinical Services
Department of Neurology
McKnight Brain Institute
University of Florida College of Medicine
Gainesville, Florida

FRANK M. SKIDMORE, MD

Assistant Professor
Department of Neurology
University of Florida College of Medicine
Gainesville, Florida
Director, Movement Disorders Clinic
North Florida/South Georgia Veterans Health System
Gainesville, Florida

MICHAEL S. OKUN, MD

Assistant Professor
Co-Director, Movement Disorders Center
Departments of Neurology, Neurosugery, and Psychiatry
McKnight Brain Institute
University of Florida College of Medicine
Gainesville, Florida

Visit our website at www.demosmedpub.com

LIBRARY OF CONGRESS CATALOGING-IN-PUBLICATION DATA
A practical approach to movement disorders : diagnosis and medical and surgical management / Hubert H. Fernandez ... [et al.].
    p. ; cm.
  Includes bibliographical references and index.
  ISBN-13: 978-1-933864-14-3 (pbk. : alk. paper)
  ISBN-10: 1-933864-14-1 (pbk. : alk. paper)
1. Movement disorders—Handbooks, manuals, etc.   I. Fernandez, Hubert H.
  DNLM: 1. Movement Disorders--Handbooks.   WL 39 P895 2007]
  RC376.5.P73 2007
  616.8'3—dc22

                                                                    2007009355

Medicine is an ever-changing science undergoing continual development. Research and clinical experience are continually expanding our knowledge, in particular our knowledge of proper treatment and drug therapy. The authors, editors, and publisher have made every effort to ensure that all information in this book is in accordance with the state of knowledge at the time of production of the book.

Nevertheless, this does not imply or express any guarantee or responsibility on the part of the authors, editors, or publisher with respect to any dosage instructions and forms of application stated in the book. Every reader should examine carefully the package inserts accompanying each drug and check with a his physician or specialist whether the dosage schedules mentioned therein or the contraindications stated by the manufacturer differ from the statements made in this book. Such examination is particularly important with drugs that are either rarely used or have been newly released on the market. Every dosage schedule or every form of application used is entirely at the reader's own risk and responsibility. The editors and publisher welcome any reader to report to the publisher any discrepancies or inaccuracies noticed.

Special discounts on bulk quantities of Demos Medical Publishing books are available to corporations, professional associations, pharmaceutical companies, health care organizations, and other qualifying groups. For details, please contact:

Special Sales Department
Demos Medical Publishing
386 Park Avenue South, Suite 301
New York, NY 10016
Phone: 800–532–8663 or 212–683–0072
Fax: 212–683–0118
Email: orderdept@demosmedpub.com

Cover design by Aimee Davis
Manufactured in the United States of America

07 08 09 10   5 4 3 2 1

DEDICATION

This book is warmly dedicated to individuals in our lives who always believed in us and continue to have undying faith in our abilities.

To our proud parents, Henry and Julie Fernandez, Ramon and Juanita Rodriguez, Francis and Dorethe Skidmore, Jack and Rosalind Okun. To our loving wives, Cecilia Fernandez, Jennifer Rodriguez, Tracy Skidmore, and Leslie Okun; and our dear patients at the University of Florida Movement Disorders Center.

CONTENTS

CONTENTS

PREFACE

While several comprehensive textbooks on movement disorders exist, most are lengthy, thick, hard-bound books that make it less useful for the busy, practicing clinician who often needs a quick guide for the diagnostic approach and therapy for various movement disorders. There are a few practical, therapeutic handbooks on Parkinson's disease but there are none that includes the other types of movement disorders (such as chorea, dystonia, myoclonus, and ataxia).

To fill this need, we created a handy, paper-bound, fit-in-your coat pocket, practical, yet authoritative, symptom-based guide to all the types of movement disorders for the practicing clinician. We used an expanded outline bulleted point format with emphasis on clinical presentation, diagnosis, workup, and management. This handbook should provide the clinician with a quick, yet comprehensive, guide to the assessment, workup, and management of the most common types of movement disorders encountered in clinical practice.

We realize that much is expected of today's clinician. Treatment now goes beyond pharmacotherapy. Thus, this handbook is divided into three parts: (1) medical, (2) surgical, and (3) other nonpharmacologic approaches. The first section, on the medical approach, is symptom based, rather than disease based, to provide a starting point for the clinician who is presented with a movement disorder but not with a known diagnosis. Unique to this book is the second section which provides the key concepts of surgical therapy not only for Parkinson's disease but also for other movement disorders. The last section acknowledges the need for a comprehensive approach that includes nutritional, physical, occupational, speech, and swallowing therapy.

It is our hope that this handbook makes the assessment and treatment of the most common movement disorders less intimidating and more rewarding for the busy clinician.

Hubert H. Fernandez, MD
Ramon L. Rodriguez, MD
Frank M. Skidmore, MD
Michael S. Okun, MD

1

GETTING STARTED:
THE PHENOMENOLOGY OF
MOVEMENT DISORDERS

Movement disorders can be defined as neurologic syndromes in which there is either an excess of movement (*hyperkinetic movements*) or a paucity of voluntary or automatic movements (*hypokinetic movements*) (Figure 1.1). Movement disorders are usually unrelated to weakness or to spasticity.

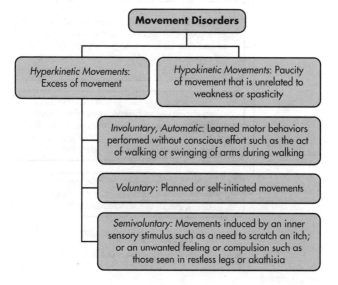

Figure 1.1
Classification of movement disorders.

Hypokinesia (decreased amplitude of movement) is sometimes called bradykinesia (slowness of movement) and akinesia (loss of movement). *Parkinsonism* is the most common cause of hypokinetic movements, but there are other less common causes of hypokinetic syndromes such as *cataplexy* and *drop attacks, catatonia, hypothyroid slowness, rigidity*, and *stiff muscles* (Figure 1.2).

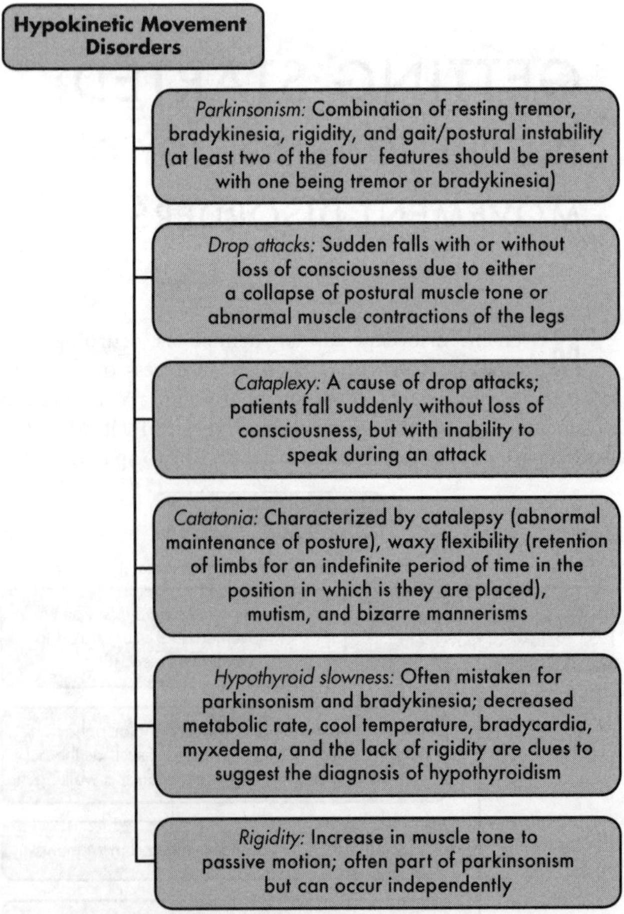

Hypokinetic Movement Disorders

Parkinsonism: Combination of resting tremor, bradykinesia, rigidity, and gait/postural instability (at least two of the four features should be present with one being tremor or bradykinesia)

Drop attacks: Sudden falls with or without loss of consciousness due to either a collapse of postural muscle tone or abnormal muscle contractions of the legs

Cataplexy: A cause of drop attacks; patients fall suddenly without loss of consciousness, but with inability to speak during an attack

Catatonia: Characterized by catalepsy (abnormal maintenance of posture), waxy flexibility (retention of limbs for an indefinite period of time in the position in which is they are placed), mutism, and bizarre mannerisms

Hypothyroid slowness: Often mistaken for parkinsonism and bradykinesia; decreased metabolic rate, cool temperature, bradycardia, myxedema, and the lack of rigidity are clues to suggest the diagnosis of hypothyroidism

Rigidity: Increase in muscle tone to passive motion; often part of parkinsonism but can occur independently

Figure 1.2
Classification of hypokinetic movement disorders.

Hyperkinesias have also been called dyskinesias or abnormal involuntary movements. The six major categories of hyperkinetic movement disorders are: *restless legs, tremor, chorea, dystonia, myoclonus,* and *tics* (Figure 1.3). However, there exist other less common hyperkinetic movement disorders such as akathisia, hemifacial spasm, hyperekplexia, myokimia, periodic leg movements of sleep, painful legs moving toes, alien limb, belly dancer's dyskinesia, and stereotypy (Figure 1.4).

These hyperkinetic disorders can be involuntary, automatic (i.e., learned motor behaviors performed without conscious effort such as the act of walking or swinging of arms during walking), voluntary (planned or self-initiated), semivoluntary (induced by an inner sensory stimulus such as a need to scratch an itch, or an unwanted feeling or compulsion—such as those seen in restless legs or akathisia).

Most, but not all, movement disorders result from some element of basal ganglia dysfunction—what is sometimes termed "extrapyramidal disorders." Movement disorders can also result from injury to the cerebral cortex, cerebellum, brainstem, spinal cord, peripheral nerve, and other central and peripheral nervous system elements.

PREVALENCE OF MOVEMENT DISORDERS

Movement disorders are quite common. Prior to the recognition of restless legs syndrome (RLS), essential tremor (ET) used to be the most common movement disorder. The estimated prevalence rates of the most common movement disorders per 100,000 of the general population[1] are given in Table 1.1.

TYPES OF HYPOKINETIC MOVEMENTS

Parkinsonism, the most recognized form of hypokinesia, accounts for approximately half of all hypokinetic movement disorders. It is manifested by any combination of four cardinal features: resting tremor, bradykinesia (slowness in movement), rigidity (stiffness), and gait/postural instability. At least two of these features need to be present with one being resting tremor or bradykinesia before the diagnosis of parkinsonism is made.

- There are several causes of parkinsonism: primary, secondary, parkinson-plus, and heredodegenerative disorders.

    - *Primary parkinsonism* (Parkinson's disease, PD) refers to a progressive disorder of unclear etiology, and the

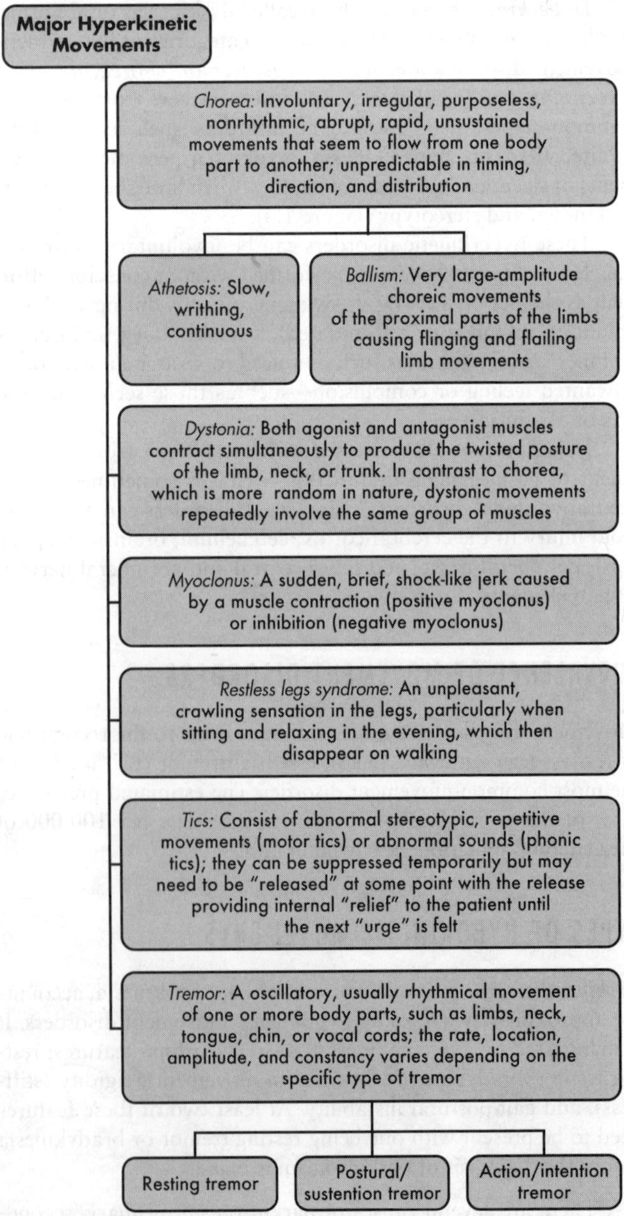

Major Hyperkinetic Movements

Chorea: Involuntary, irregular, purposeless, nonrhythmic, abrupt, rapid, unsustained movements that seem to flow from one body part to another; unpredictable in timing, direction, and distribution

Athetosis: Slow, writhing, continuous

Ballism: Very large-amplitude choreic movements of the proximal parts of the limbs causing flinging and flailing limb movements

Dystonia: Both agonist and antagonist muscles contract simultaneously to produce the twisted posture of the limb, neck, or trunk. In contrast to chorea, which is more random in nature, dystonic movements repeatedly involve the same group of muscles

Myoclonus: A sudden, brief, shock-like jerk caused by a muscle contraction (positive myoclonus) or inhibition (negative myoclonus)

Restless legs syndrome: An unpleasant, crawling sensation in the legs, particularly when sitting and relaxing in the evening, which then disappear on walking

Tics: Consist of abnormal stereotypic, repetitive movements (motor tics) or abnormal sounds (phonic tics); they can be suppressed temporarily but may need to be "released" at some point with the release providing internal "relief" to the patient until the next "urge" is felt

Tremor: A oscillatory, usually rhythmical movement of one or more body parts, such as limbs, neck, tongue, chin, or vocal cords; the rate, location, amplitude, and constancy varies depending on the specific type of tremor

Resting tremor

Postural/ sustention tremor

Action/intention tremor

Figure 1.3

Classification of major hyperkinetic movement disorders.

Other Hyperkinetic Movements

Akathisia: The inability to remain still because of an inner sense of restlessness

Hyperekplexia: Abnormal excessive startle in response to sudden unexpected stimulus. It occurs in three conditions: startle disease (familial or sporadic), startle epilepsy, and jumping Frenchmen of Maine syndrome

Hemifacial spasms: Unilateral contraction of facial muscles involving the eyelids, cheek, and corner of the mouth

Myokimia: Visible rippling movements from continuous muscle contractions

Stereotypy: Involuntary (or involuntary) coordinated, patterned, repetitive, rhythmic, purposeless, but seemingly purposeful, or ritualistic movement, posture, or utterance

Alien limb: A feeling of "foreignness" about movements of the affected limb or a lack of recognition of the movement of the affected limb

Periodic leg movements of sleep: Nocturnal myoclonus; repetitive stereotypical extension of the big toe, the ankle, knee, and hip by flexion after the toe has extended; occur in clusters throughout sleep

Painful legs moving toes: Continuous, stereotypical, and flexion-extension or adduction-abduction movements of the toes; there is no subjective; sensory symptoms can be mild or excruciatingly painful

FIGURE 1.4

Descriptions of other hyperkinetic movement disorder phenomenologies.

TABLE 1.1
The Estimated Prevalence Rates of the Most Common
Movement Disorders per 100,000 of the General Population

Restless legs	9800
Essential tremor	415
Parkinson's disease	187
Tourette's syndrome	29–1052
Primary torsion dystonia	33
Hemifacial spasm	7.4–14.5
Blepharospasm	13.3
Hereditary ataxia	6
Huntington's disease	2–12
Wilson's disease	3
Progressive supranuclear palsy	2–6.4
Multiple system atrophy	4.4

diagnosis is often made by excluding other causes of parkinsonism. For this reason, it is also called "idiopathic" PD. It is probably the most common type of parkinsonism encountered by a neurologist.

■ *Secondary parkinsonism* refers to disorders with an identifiable cause such as drug-induced parkinsonism (from intake of dopamine receptor–blocking agents such as antipsychotic and anti-emetic drugs), or parkinsonism resulting from a stroke, infection, or tumor in a region of the basal ganglia.

■ *Parkinson-plus syndromes* are also progressive neurodegenerative disorders with parkinsonism as their main, but not the only, feature. Examples of parkinson-plus disorders are progressive supranuclear palsy (with early dementia, vertical gaze palsy, and early, frequent falls), multiple systems atrophy (with lack of tremor, more prominent cerebellar features such as ataxia and incoordination, significant autonomic dysfunction such as urinary incontinence, erectile dysfunction, or orthostatic hypotension), and corticobasoganglionic degeneration or corticobasal degeneration (presenting with early dementia, cortical sensory loss, apraxia, limb dystonia, and "alien limb phenomenon"—where the limb performs autonomous movements).

■ Finally, other neurodegenerative disorders can also present with parkinsonism. The main difference between this group (compared to the parkinson-plus) of disorders is that parkinsonism is not their most prominent feature. For example, Alzheimer's disease is primarily a neurodegenerative disorder of memory dysfunction but parkinsonism can occur at the later stages of the illness.

OTHER HYPOKINETIC MOVEMENTS

■ *Drop attacks* can be defined as sudden falls with or without loss of consciousness due to either a collapse of postural muscle tone or abnormal muscle contractions of the legs. About two-thirds of the cases of drop attacks are of unknown etiology. Known causes include epilepsy, myoclonus, startle reactions, and structural CNS lesions. Syncope is the most common nonneurologic cause.

■ *Cataplexy* is another cause of symptomatic drop attack. Patients fall suddenly without loss of consciousness, but with inability to speak during an attack. There is often a preceding trigger, usually laughter or a sudden emotional stimulus. It is usually one of the four cardinal features of narcolepsy (which also include excessive sleepiness, sleep paralysis, and hypnagogic hallucinations).

■ *Catatonia* is actually a syndrome, not a specific diagnosis, that is characterized by catalepsy (development of fixed postures), waxy flexibility (retention of limbs for an indefinite period of time in the position in which they are placed), mutism, and bizarre mannerisms. Patients remain in one position for hours and move exceedingly slow to commands, but when moving spontaneously (such as scratching themselves), they do it quickly. Catatonia is classically a feature of schizophrenia, but can occur with severe depression, hysterical disorders, and even in organic brain disease.

■ *Hypothyroid slowness* can be mistaken for parkinsonism and bradykinesia. But additional clues such as decreased metabolic rate, cool temperature, bradycardia, myxedema, and the lack of rigidity, represent clues suggesting the diagnosis.

■ *Rigidity* is characterized by an increase in muscle tone with passive motion. It is distinguished from spasticity (a sign of corticospinal tract/pyramidal lesion) in that it is present equally in all directions of the passive movement, and it is not velocity dependent, and therefore it does not exhibit the "clasp-knife" phenomenon). Rigidity is often present with parkinsonism but can also occur independently.

TYPES OF HYPERKINETIC MOVEMENTS

- *Chorea* refers to involuntary, irregular, purposeless, non-rhythmic, abrupt, rapid, unsustained movements that seem to flow from one body part to another. They are unpredictable in timing, direction, and distribution. They can be partially suppressed, and the patient can often camouflage some of the movements by incorporating them into semipurposeful movements (termed "parakinesias"). An example of a movement disorder that presents primarily with chorea is Huntington's disease.

  - When the involuntary movements are slow, writhing, and continuous, they are sometimes called athetosis.

  - When they are very large-amplitude choreic movements of the proximal parts of the limbs causing flinging and flailing limb movements, they are referred to as ballism. Ballism is most frequently unilateral and is classically described as resulting from a lesion of the contralateral subthalamic nucleus.

  - Athetosis, chorea, and ballism may represent a continuum of one type of hyperkinetic movement disorder and are sometimes combined (choreoathetosis or chorea-ballism).

- *Dystonia*: is characterized by involuntary, sustained, patterned, and often repetitive muscle contractions of opposing muscles, causing twisting movements or abnormal postures. In contrast to chorea, which is more random in nature, dystonic movements usually, and repeatedly, involve the same group of muscles.

  - When a single body part is affected, it is called focal dystonia. Examples of focal dystonia include blepharospasm (dystonia of the eyelids), spasmodic torticollis (cervical or neck dystonia), spasmodic dystonia (vocal cords), and writer's cramp (hand dystonia).

  - Involvement of two or more contiguous regions of the body is referred to as segmental dystonia.

- *Generalized dystonia* refers to involvement of the trunk, legs, and other body parts. Idiopathic torsional dystonia, more common among Ashkenazi Jews, is an example of an autosomal dominant disorder (with incomplete penetrance) that begins in childhood as a focal or segmental dystonia and may later generalize to include the entire body.

- *Myoclonus* is a sudden, brief, shock-like jerk caused by a muscle contraction (positive myoclonus) or inhibition (negative myoclonus).

  - The most common form of negative myoclonus is asterixis from hepatic or renal impairment. The causes of myoclonus are quite diverse and may vary from epileptic syndromes, to drug side effects, metabolic disturbances, and central nervous system (CNS) lesions.

- *Restless legs syndrome* (RLS) is a syndrome characterized by a desire to move the legs. The updated standardized clinical criteria for the diagnosis of RLS by the International RLS Study Group are as follows:

  - A desire to move the limbs (with or without paresthesia), and the arms may be involved.

  - The urge to move or the unpleasant sensation improves with activity, and symptoms are worse with rest or inactivity.

  - The urge to move or the unpleasant sensations are partially or totally relieved with movement.

  - The symptoms have a circadian variation, occurring most often in the evening or at night when the patient lies down. The patient often describes an unpleasant, crawling sensation in the legs, particularly when sitting and relaxing in the evening, which then disappear on walking.

    - RLS is a very common illness. There are two distinct types: primary (idiopathic) or secondary.

      - The majority of individuals with primary RLS have a positive family history. It has a high concordance in monozygotic twins. An autosomal dominant mode of inheritance has been proposed.

      - Secondary RLS is often associated with iron deficiency anemia, pregnancy, end-stage renal disease, and certain medications such as antidepressants and dopamine-blocking agents.

- *Tics* consist of abnormal movements (motor tics) or abnormal sounds (phonic tics). When both types of tics are present, and occurring under the age of 21 accompanied by obsessive-compulsive features, the designation of Tourette's syndrome is commonly applied. Tics frequently vary in severity over time and can have remissions and exacerbations. Motor and phonic tics can be simple or complex. Most of the time tics are repetitive. They can be suppressed temporarily but will need to be "released" at some point providing internal "relief" to the patient until the next "urge" is felt. Examples include shoulder shrug, head jerk, blink, twitch of the nose, touching other people, head shaking with shoulder shrugging, kicking of the legs, obscene gesturing, grunting, or throat clearing.

- *Tremor* is an oscillatory, usually rhythmical, to and fro regular movement affecting one or more body parts, such as limbs, neck, tongue, chin, or vocal cords. The rate, location, amplitude, and constancy varies depending on the specific type of tremor. Tremors can be present at rest (resting tremor), with posture holding (postural tremor) or with action such as writing or pouring water (intention or kinetic tremor).

  - Resting tremor, for example, while on its own is a hyperkinetic movement, is often part of a hypokinetic movement disorder: parkinsonism.

  - When tremor occurs mostly with action or intention, the most common cause is benign essential tremor—a nonprogressive disorder which can either be hereditary (usually autosomal dominant) or sporadic.

  - When the tremor frequency is rapid and most prominent with posture holding, it can be a manifestation of enhanced physiologic tremor. Conditions that "enhance" the silent tremor (or sometimes referred to as a physiologic tremor which is present in all humans) include hyperthyroidism, anxiety, hypoglycemia, and medications such as steroids and antiasthma agents such as terbutaline and albuterol.

REFERENCE

1. Schrag A. Epidemiology of movement disorders. In: Jankovic J, Tolosa E, eds. Parkinson's Disease and Movement Disorders, 4th ed. Philadelphia: Lippincott, Williams & Wilkins, 2002:73–89.

2

THE "DANCING" PATIENT

PHENOMENOLOGY

Chorea, athetosis, and ballism generally represent a continuum of involuntary, hyperkinetic movement disorders.

Chorea consists of involuntary, continuous, abrupt, rapid, brief, unsustained, irregular movements that flow randomly from one body part to another.

Ballism is a form of forceful, flinging, high-amplitude, coarse chorea; ballism and chorea are often interrelated and may occur in the same patient.

Athetosis is a slow form of chorea and consists of writhing movements resembling dystonia, but unlike dystonia, the movements are not sustained, patterned, repetitive or painful.

Akathisia is characterized by a feeling of inner restlessness and jitteriness with inability to sit or stand still.

Restless legs syndrome is a symptom complex of discomfort in the legs (or arm) that is characteristically relieved by movements.

CHOREA
Clinical Features

- Patients can partially or temporarily suppress the chorea.

- *Parakinesia is* the act of "camouflaging" some of the movements by incorporating them into semipurposeful activities.

- *Motor impersistence* is the inability to maintain voluntary contraction; e.g., milkmaid's grip, tongue protrusion.

- Chorea must be differentiated from pseudochoreoathetosis (chorea or athetosis secondary to a proprioceptive defect).

- Chorea may be a manifestation of a primary neurologic disorder (such as Huntington's disease) or as a complication of systemic, toxic, or other disorders.

Differential Diagnoses (Figure 2.1)

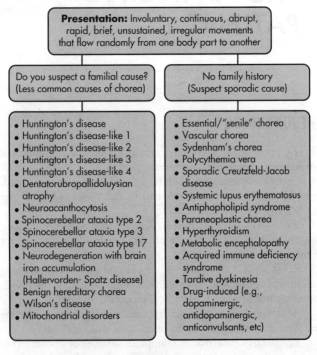

Presentation: Involuntary, continuous, abrupt, rapid, brief, unsustained, irregular movements that flow randomly from one body part to another

Do you suspect a familial cause? (Less common causes of chorea)

- Huntington's disease
- Huntington's disease-like 1
- Huntington's disease-like 2
- Huntington's disease-like 3
- Huntington's disease-like 4
- Dentatorubropallidoluysian atrophy
- Neuroacanthocytosis
- Spinocerebellar ataxia type 2
- Spinocerebellar ataxia type 3
- Spinocerebellar ataxia type 17
- Neurodegeneration with brain iron accumulation (Hallervorden- Spatz disease)
- Benign hereditary chorea
- Wilson's disease
- Mitochondrial disorders

No family history (Suspect sporadic cause)

- Essential/"senile" chorea
- Vascular chorea
- Sydenham's chorea
- Polycythemia vera
- Sporadic Creutzfeld-Jacob disease
- Systemic lupus erythematosus
- Antiphopholipid syndrome
- Paraneoplastic chorea
- Hyperthyroidism
- Metabolic encephalopathy
- Acquired immune deficiency syndrome
- Tardive dyskinesia
- Drug-induced (e.g., dopaminergic, antidopaminergic, anticonvulsants, etc)

FIGURE 2.1
Differential diagnosis of chorea.

CLASSIFICATION

Inherited Causes

1. *Huntington's disease* (HD) is an autosomal dominant neurodegenerative disorder (therefore, each child of an affected

parent has a 50% chance of developing the disease) due to an abnormal expansion of IT-15 gene on chromosome 4, which encodes for the protein Huntingtin.

- Most people develop HD between 30 and 54 years old, but it can manifest as early as 4 years old and as late as 80 years.

- It is a CAG repeat disease: normal is 10–35; indeterminate: 36–39; definite: 40 or more.

- Triad of motor, cognitive, and psychiatric symptoms.

- Motor: impairment of involuntary (chorea) and voluntary movements; reduced manual dexterity, slurred speech, swallowing difficulties, balance problems, and falls; parkinsonism; dystonia in the young.

  - When treating chorea, consider non-drug interventions first.

  - Pharmacologic treatment for chorea may worsen other aspects of the movement disorder, cognition, or mood.

  - Chorea may diminish over time, reducing the need for treatment.

- Cognitive: initially by loss of speed and flexibility; later become more global.

- Psychiatric: depression (most common), mania, obsessive-compulsive disorder, irritability, anxiety, agitation, impulsivity, apathy, social withdrawal.

  - Ask about substance abuse.

  - Always ask about suicide.

- Diagnosis: clinical presentation, family history, and genetic testing (genetic counseling is required for asymptomatic individuals with a family history).

  - Always disclose results in person, with a patient's relative, caregiver, or friend present.

  - Prenatal testing (as early as 8–10 weeks) is possible. A nondisclosing prenatal test, which determines only whether or not the fetus received a chromosome from the affected grand-parent, without determining whether the fetus or the at-risk parent actually caries the gene, is possible but requires samples from several individuals.

- Nonpharmacologic approaches to some functional difficulties and behavioral dysfunction in Huntington's disease (Table 2.1).

TABLE 2.1
Helpful Tips on Functional and Behavioral Problems in HD

Problem	Solution
Swallowing difficulties	Eat slowly and without distractions.
	Prepare foods with appropriate size and texture.
	May need to supervise eating.
	All caregivers should know the Heimlich maneuver.
Communication tips	Allow the patient enough time to answer the question.
	Offer cues and prompts to get the patient started.
	Give choices rather than open-ended questions.
	Break the task or instructions down into small steps.
	Use visual cues to demonstrate what you are saying.
	Alphabet boards, yes-no cards, other devices for more advanced stages.
Disorganized thought process	Rely on routines, they are easier to initiate.
	Make lists which help organize tasks.
	Prompt each activity with external cues.
	Offer limited choices instead of open-ended questions.
	Use short sentences with one to two pieces of information.
Impulsivity	A predictable daily schedule can reduce confusion, fear, outbursts.
	It is possible that a behavior is a response to something that needs your attention.
	Stay calm.
	Let the patient know that yelling is not the best way to get your attention.
	Hurtful and embarrassing statements are generally not intentional. Be sensitive to the patient's efforts to apologize or his show of remorse afterward.
	Do not badger the person after the fact.

TABLE 2.1 (cont.)

Problem	Solution
Irritability and temper outbursts	Try to keep the environment as calm as possible.
	Speak in a low, soft voice. Keep your hand gestures quiet.
	Avoid confrontations.
	Redirect the patient away from the source of anger.
	Respond diplomatically, acknowledging the patients irritability as a symptom of frustration.

Source: Adapted from reference 1.

2. *Huntington-like syndromes* (Table 2.2)

3. *Inherited "paroxysmal" choreas* (Table 2.3) (See Chapter 6 for details.)

Sporadic Causes

1. Essential chorea is an adult-onset, nonprogressive chorea without family history or other symptoms suggestive of HD and without evidence of striatal atrophy. "Senile chorea" is a type of essential chorea in which the usual onset is after age 60, but without dementia or psychiatric disturbance.

2. In infectious chorea, acute manifestations of bacterial meningitis, encephalitis, tuberculous meningitis, aseptic meningitis, HIV encephalitis, and toxoplasmosis have been described.

3. Postinfectious/autoimmune choreas include:

■ Sydenham's disease (St. Vitus' dance): Associated with infection with group A streptococci; chorea may be delayed for 6 months or longer; distribution is often asymmetrical; may be accompanied by arthritis, carditis, irritability, emotional lability, obsessive-compulsive disorder (OCD), anxiety; elevated titers of antistreptolysin (ASO).

■ Systemic lupus erythematosus (SLE): Associated with antiphospholipid syndrome (characterized by migraine, chorea, venous or arterial thrombosis); positive antiphospholipid antibodies

TABLE 2.2
Summary of Huntington-like Syndromes

Disease	MOI	Chromosome	Gene	Triplet repeat	Protein	Features
Huntington-like disease 1[2]	AD	20p	HDL1	No		Similar to HD-like 2 but seizures can occur.
Huntington-like disease 2[3]	AD	16q23	HDL2	CTG/CAG	Junctophilin-3	Onset in the fourth decade; chorea, dystonia, parkinsonism, dysarthria, hyperreflexia, gait abnormality, psychiatric symptoms, weight loss dementia; acanthocytosis is common; predominantly African Americans
Huntington-like disease 3	AR	4p15.3		No		Begins at 3–4 years old; chorea, ataxia, gait disorder, spasticity, seizures, mutism, dementia
Neuroacanth-ocytosis[4]	AR, some AD or sporadic	9q21-22	CHAC	No	Chorein	After HD, most common hereditary chorea; begins third to fourth decade, lip and tongue biting, orolingual dystonia, motor and phonic tics, generalized chorea, parkinsonism, vertical ophthalmoparesis, seizures, cognitive and personality changes, dysphagia, dysarthria, amyotrophy, areflexia, axonal neuropathy, elevated CPK; acanthocytes on peripheral smear
McLeod syndrome[5]	X recessive	X	XK	No	KX	Form of neuroacanthocytosis; depression, bipolar and personality disorders, chorea, vocalizations, seizures, hemolysis, liver disease, high CK; usually no lip biting or dysphagia
Benign hereditary chorea[6]	AD	14q13.1-21.1		No		Nonprogressive chorea of childhood onset; slight motor delay, ataxia, may be self-limiting

	MOI	Locus	Gene	Repeat	Protein	Notes
SCA 2	AD	12q23-24.1	SCA2	CAG	Ataxin-2	Commercially available gene testing
SCA 3	AD	14q32.1	SCA3	CAG	Ataxin-3	Machado-Joseph disease; Azorean descent; parkinsonism, dystonia, chorea, neuropathy, ataxia; commercially available testing
SCA 17	AD	6q27	SCA 17	CAG	TATA-binding protein	Commercially available gene testing
DRPLA[7]	AD	12		CAG	JNK	More commonly reported in Japan > Europe, Africans, southern U.S. (Haw River syndrome); starts in the fourth decade; combination of choreoathetosis, dystonia, tremor, parkinsonism, dementia
Neurodegeneration with brain iron accumulation (NBIA) type 1 (formerly Hallervorden-Spatz disease)[8]	AR	20p112.3-13	PANK-2	No	Pantothenate kinase	Childhood-onset progressive rigidity, dystonia, choreoathetosis, spasticity, optic nerve atrophy, dementia, acanthocytosis; "eye of the tiger" MRI abnormality
Wilson's disease	AR	13q14.3	ATB7B	No	Cu-ATPase	May present with tremor, parkinsonism, dystonia, chorea; usually before age 50. See also Chapter 6.

AD, autosomal dominant; AR, autosomal recessive; CK, creatine kinase; CPK, creatine phosphokinase; DRPLA, dentatorubropallidoluysian atrophy; MOI, method of inheritance; MRI, magnetic resonance imaging; NBIA, Neurodegeneration of the brain with iron accumulation; SCA, spinocerebellar ataxia.

TABLE 2.3
Summary of Features of Major Causes of Paroxysmal Dyskinesias

	PKD	PND	PED
Male/female ratio	4:1	3:2	Unclear
Age of onset	5–15	Less than 5 years	2–0
Inheritance	AD or sporadic	AD or sporadic	AD
Duration of attacks	<5 minutes	Several minutes-hours	5–30 minutes
Frequency	Very frequent, 100/day to 1/month	Occasional, 3/day to 2/year	1/day to 1/month
Asymmetry	common	Less common	
Ability to suppress attacks	Able	Able	
Precipitating factors	Sudden movement, startle, hyperventilation, fatigue, stress	Alcohol, caffeine, exercise, excitement	Prolonged exercise, stress, caffeine, fatigue
Associated features	Dystonia, chorea, epilepsy	Chorea, dystonia, ataxia	Dystonia, chorea
Treatment	Phenytoin, carbamazepine, barbiturates, acetazolamide	Clonazepam, oxazepam	

AD, autosomal dominant; PED, paroxysmal exertional dyskinesia; PKD, paroxysmal kinesogenic dyskinesia; PND, paroxysmal nonkinesogenic dyskinesia.

(APLA) and anti-cardiolipin antibodies; spontaneous abortions, arthralgias, Raynaud's phenomenon, digital infarctions, transient ischemic attacks (TIAs), cerebrovascular accidents (CVAs).

■ Chorea gravidarum: May occur with recurrence of SLE or Sydenham's disease during pregnancy.

4. Postpump chorea is a sequela of cardiac surgery (for congenital heart disease) in children; associated with prolonged time on the pump, deep hypothermia, circulatory arrest; some respond to dopamine receptor–blocking agents.

5. Although polycythemia vera is more common in men, it is more often associated with chorea when seen in women; facial erythrosis or splenomegaly may be present; onset is usually after

TABLE 2.4
Drugs Reported to Cause Tardive Syndromes

Amoxapine (tricyclic antidepressant)
Chlorpromazine
Chlorprothixene
Cinnarizine (calcium channel blocker)
Clebopride
Clozapine (?)
Droperidol
Flunarizine (calcium channel blocker)
Fluphenazine
Haloperidol
Loxapine
Mesoridazine
Metoclopramide
Molindone
Olanzapine
Perazine
Pimozide
Prochlorperazine
Quetiapine (?)
Remoxipride
Risperidone
Sulpiride
Tiapride
Trifluoperazine
Triflupromazine
Thioridazine
Thiothixene
Veralipride

50 years, and the chorea is often bilateral and symmetrical; treatment is with both reduction of hyperviscosity and antidopaminergic drugs.

6. Vascular chorea has been described in congophilic angiopathy and other types of strokes.

7. Paraneoplastic chorea is mostly associated with CRMP-5 or CV2 antibodies (commercially available testing).

8. There are two types of drug-induced choreas:

■ Those occurring acutely with, e.g., dopaminergic or antidopaminergic drugs and anticonvulsants.

■ Tardive chorea in which stereotypic orobuccolingual dyskinesia occurs after chronic exposure to dopamine receptor–blocking agents (Table 2.4).

9. The metabolic etiologies of chorea, which may be asymmetrical, are:

■ Hypocalcemia and hypercalcemia

■ Hypoglycemia and hyperglycemia

■ Hyperthyroidism

■ Hyponatremia and hypernatremia

■ Hypomagnesemia

■ Hypoparathyroidism and hyperparathyroidsim

■ Liver disease (acquired hepatocerebral degeneration)

10. Although rare, any movement disorder can be associated with multiple sclerosis. Chorea and/or tremor may be the most common movement disorder presentation. Ballism has also been reported.

Diagnostic Workup (Figure 2.2):

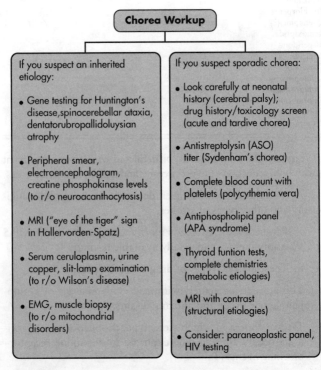

Chorea Workup

If you suspect an inherited etiology:

• Gene testing for Huntington's disease,spinocerebellar ataxia, dentatorubropallidoluysian atrophy

• Peripheral smear, electroencephalogram, creatine phosphokinase levels (to r/o neuroacanthocytosis)

• MRI ("eye of the tiger" sign in Hallervorden-Spatz)

• Serum ceruloplasmin, urine copper, slit-lamp examination (to r/o Wilson's disease)

• EMG, muscle biopsy (to r/o mitochondrial disorders)

If you suspect sporadic chorea:

• Look carefully at neonatal history (cerebral palsy); drug history/toxicology screen (acute and tardive chorea)

• Antistreptolysin (ASO) titer (Sydenham's chorea)

• Complete blood count with platelets (polycythemia vera)

• Antiphospholipid panel (APA syndrome)

• Thyroid funtion tests, complete chemistries (metabolic etiologies)

• MRI with contrast (structural etiologies)

• Consider: paraneoplastic panel, HIV testing

FIGURE 2.2
Initial workup for a patient presenting with chorea.

Treatment (Table 2.5):

TABLE 2.5
Medications Used to Suppress Chorea

Class	Medication	Starting dose (mg/d)	Maximum dose (mg/d)	Adverse events
Neuroleptics	Haloperidol	0.5–1	6–8	Sedation, parkinsonism, dystonia, akathisia, hypotension, constipation, dry mouth, weight gain, confusion
	Fluphenazine	0.5–1	6–8	Same
	Risperidone	0.5–1	6	Same
	Thiothixene	1–2	6	Same
	Thioridazine	10	100	Same
	Clozapine	12.5	600	Less parkinsonism but rare agranulocytosis requires weekly complete blood count monitoring for first 6 months and every 2 weeks thereafter
	Quetiapine	25	800	Less parkinsonism
Benzodiazepines	Clonazepam	0.5	4	Sedation, ataxia, apathy, withdrawal seizures
	Diazepam	1.25	20	Same
N-methyl-D-aspartate antagonist	Amantadine	100	400	Hallucinations, confusion, leg swelling, livido reticularis; anticholinergic effects
Dopamine receptor–blocking agents	Reserpine	0.1	3	Hypotension, sedation, depression
	Tetrabenazine	25	100	Less hypotension, need to order from Canada or United Kingdom

1. The first step is always to try to identify the underlying etiology.

2. Dopamine receptor–blocking agents (atypical neuroleptics preferred over typicals if possible), if the chorea is disrupting quality of life.

3. Reserpine.

4. Tetrabenazine.

5. Consider divalproex (Depakote).

6. Anticoagulation, immunosuppressants, and plasmapheresis have been used with variable success in autoimmune choreas; consider steroids.

7. Consider stereotactic surgery for severe and disabling cases of chorea or ballism.[9] See Chapter 9.

8. Tardive dyskinesia (TD):

- The severity of the tardive syndrome and the absolute need for neuroleptic therapy often dictate the treatment approach for this group of disorders.

- Continuing to use drugs known to cause tardive phenomena is not the best approach and increasing the dose may be a temporary solution.

- Because a substantial fraction of TD patients may remit if kept off dopamine, a receptor–blocking agent (DRBA), the first choice is to avoid any antipsychotic drug. When this is not possible, as is usually the case, clozapine is the best choice but logistically difficult to use (requires blood counts).

- To suppress mild TD, low doses of benzodiazepine or vitamin E, in addition to switching to clozapine or quetiapine, might be helpful.

- For moderate to severe TD, dopamine depleters such as tetrabenazine or reserpine may be the most effective agents.

- Only as a last resort, for persistent, disabling, and treatment-resistant TD, should neuroleptics be resumed to treat TD in the absence of active psychosis.

BALLISM

Damage to the subthalamic nucleus and the pallidosubthalamic pathways usually play a critical role in the underlying causes of ballism, although other structures have been implicated/described (especially the thalamus).

Etiology

1. When caused by a hemorrhagic or ischemic stroke, ballism is often preceded by hemiparesis.

2. Also described in anterior parietal stroke.

3. Less common causes: abscess, arteriovenous malformation, cerebral trauma, hyperosmotic hyperglycemia, multiple sclerosis, tumor, BG strokes or calcification, encephalitis, and vasculitis

Prognosis and Treatment

1. Prognosis for spontaneous remission may be good

2. DRPAs (haloperidol, chlorpromazine, pimozide, and atypical neuroleptics) are the most frequently used.

3. Reserpine and tetrabenazine may be considered.

4. Depakote and clonazepam have been reported to improve ballism.

5. For violent, treatment-refractory ballism, ventrolateral thalamotomy has been described, and DBS may be an option.

ATHETOSIS

Chorea often evolves to athetosis and vice versa, or they coexist (choreoathetosis):

- Most often accompanies cerebral palsy; other cases are due to errors of metabolism and include acidurias, lipidosis, and Lesch-Nyhan syndrome.

- Treatment: Usually does not respond to therapy; try levodopa first (to rule out dopamine-responsive dystonia), then anticholinergic drugs (such as benztropine or trihexyphenidyl, similar to the treatment of dystonia).

AKATHISIA AND RESTLESS LEGS

Akathisia is characterized by a feeling of inner restlessness and jitteriness with inability to sit or stand still.

- Patients subjectively complain of feeling fidgety and nervous, which is often objectively manifested by complex stereotypical movements.

- Subjectively, the most common complaint is the inability to keep the legs still, but patients may also describe a vague inner tension, emotional unease, or anxiety.

- Objectively, patients are seen rocking from foot to foot, walking in place, shifting weight while sitting, and occasionally grunting, moaning, or trunk rocking.

- Depending on the timing of its appearance, akathisia may be subclassified as acute or chronic.

  - Chronic akathisia is further subdivided into that occurring early in the course of neuroleptic therapy but remains persistent, acute persistent akathisia, and that occurring with long-term therapy, tardive akathisia.

  - It is often difficult to distinguish between these two subtypes of chronic akathisia because of the imprecise information about the onset of akathisia relative to neuroleptic initiation.

- Tardive akathisia and dystonia are the most distressing and disabling of the tardive syndromes. Therefore, the offending DRBA should be stopped if possible. Unfortunately, most reports on treatment do not distinguish between acute and tardive akathisia and probably refer more to acute akathisia.

  - Anticholinergic drugs are usually ineffective. Unlike acute akathisia, beta blockers do not have good efficacy in treating tardive akathisia.

  - Reports on opiates are conflicting.

  - Reserpine and tetrabenazine may be considered.

  - Electroconvulsive therapy can be effective for intractable akathisia.

Restless legs syndrome (RLS) is a common sensorimotor disorder.

- Recent studies suggest a prevalence between 3 and 15% in the general population, greater in women, and increasing prevalence with age.

- Because the syndrome has only recently been recognized, many individuals go undiagnosed and untreated.

- The updated standardized clinical criteria for the diagnosis of RLS by the International RLS Study Group[10] are:

  - A desire to move the limbs (with or without paresthesia), and the arms may be involved.

- The urge to move, or the unpleasant sensation improves with activity, and symptoms are worse with rest or inactivity.

- The urge to move, or the unpleasant sensations are partially or totally relieved with movement.

- The symptoms have a circadian variation, occurring most often in the evening or at night when the patient lies down.

- There are two distinct types of RLS: primary (idiopathic) and secondary.

  - The majority of individuals with primary RLS have a positive family history. It has a high concordance in monozygotic twins. An autosomal dominant mode of inheritance has been proposed.

  - Secondary RLS is often associated with iron deficiency anemia, pregnancy, end-stage renal disease, and certain medications such as antidepressants and dopamine-blocking agents.

- Possible mechanisms of primary RLS pathophysiology include abnormal iron metabolism and functional alterations in central dopaminergic neurotransmitter systems.

- Nonpharmacologic treatment of RLS includes improving sleep hygiene, avoiding alcohol and caffeine, and moderate exercise daily.

  - Treatment of secondary RLS requires discontinuing offending medications and correcting iron deficiency.

  - Dopaminergic medications have the greatest efficacy in RLS.

  - Low-dose levodopa is effective but can cause augmentation (i.e., the occurrence of more severe symptoms that develop earlier in the evening), rebound (i.e., recurrence of symptoms in the early morning hours), and tolerance. Dopamine agonists are less likely to cause augmentation; however, tolerance may develop, sometimes quickly.

  - Gabapentin is the second-line therapy for those unable to tolerate dopaminergic agents.

  - Opioids may be tried as third-line therapy and benzodiazepines may provide some relief.

Painful legs and moving toes (PLMT):

■ The motor component of this syndrome is usually confined to the toes but may involve proximal parts of the legs.

■ Movements are continuous, stereotypical, flexion-extension or adduction-abduction of the toes.

■ Often disappears with sleep, relieved by rest, and hot or cold water.

■ Sensory symptoms can be mild to excruciatingly painful.

■ There is no subjective desire to move, unlike in akathisia.

■ May be associated with peripheral neuropathy or radiculopathy.

REFERENCES

1. Rosenblatt A, Ranen NG, Nance MA, Paulsen JS. A Physician's Guide to the Management of Huntington's Disease, 2nd ed. New York, Huntington's Disease Society of America, 1999.

2. Xiang F, Almqvist EW, Huq M, et al. Huntington disease-like neurodegenerative disorder maps to chromosome 20p. Am J Hum Genet 1998;63:1431–1438.

3. Walker RH, Jankovic J, O'Hearn E, Margolis RL. Phenotypic features of Huntington disease-like 2. Mov Disord 2003;18:1527–1530.

4. Spitz MC, Jankovic J, Kilian JM. Familial tic disorder, parkinsonism, motor neuron disease, and acanthocytosis—a new syndrome. Neurology 1985;35:366–377.

5. Witt TN, Danek A, Hein MU, et al. McLeod syndrome: a distinct form of neuroacanthocytosis. J Neurol 1992;239:302–306.

6. Wheeler PG, Weaver DD, Dobyns WB. Benign hereditary chorea. Pediatr Neurol 1993;9:337–340.

7. Burke JR, Wingfield MS, Lewis KE, et al. The Haw River syndrome: dentorubropallidoluysian atrophy in an African-American family. Nature Genet 1994;7: 521–524.

8. Malandrini A, Fabrizi GM, Bartalucci P, et al. Clinicopathological study of familial late infantile Hallevorden-Spatz disease: a particular form of neuroacanthocytosis. Child Nerv Syst 1996;12:155–160.

9. Krauss JK, Mundiger F. Surgical treatment of hemiballism and hemichorea. In: Krauss JK, Jankovic J, Grossman RG, eds. Surgery for Movement Disorders. Philadelphia: Lippincott Williams & Wilkins, 2000.

10. Allen RP, Picchietti D, Hening WA, et al. Restless legs syndrome: diagnostic criteria, special considerations, epidemiology: a report from the Restless Legs Syndrome Diagnosis and Epidemiology Workshop at the National Institutes of Health. Sleep Med 2003;4:101–119.

3

THE "JERKY" PATIENT

PHENOMENOLOGY

Myoclonus refers to sudden, brief, shock-like involuntary movements. Myoclonic jerks can range from mild muscular contractions that are too weak to cause discernible movement to gross jerks that can affect the entire body. The jerks can be symmetrical or asymmetrical. They usually appear to be synchronous to the clinician, but asynchronous jerking can also be seen. Myoclonus may be focal or segmental (confined to one particular region of the body), multifocal (different parts of the body affected, not necessarily at the same time), or generalized (whole body part affected in a single jerk) (Figure 3.1).

Myoclonus is often stimulus (reflex myoclonus) and activity (action myoclonus) sensitive. Sudden and unexpected noise, bright lights, or muscle stretch can trigger a myoclonic jerk. The jerks may be present at rest or may be triggered or aggravated by attempts to perform fine movements (action or intention myoclonus). Myoclonus may be rhythmic, in which case, it is usually due to a focal lesion of the spinal cord or brainstem. As a result of the rhythmicity, myoclonus may be referred to as a tremor. More typically, it is arrhythmic.

Because of the heterogeneity of the etiology of myoclonus, it is difficult to ascertain its true incidence. The only available study is from Olmstead County, Minnesota.[1] The average annual incidence was 1.3 cases per 100,000 patients. The rate increased with advancing age and was consistently higher in men.

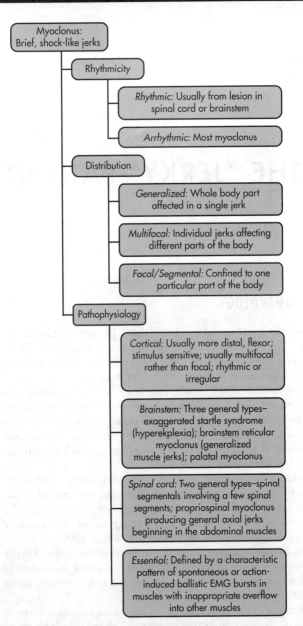

FIGURE 3.1
Classification of myoclonus.

ETIOLOGY AND CLASSIFICATION

Cortical Myoclonus

Cortical myoclonus is typically stimulus sensitive and may be precipitated by sudden loud noise or a visual stimulus.

- In cortical myoclonus, the jerks are usually more distal than proximal and more flexor than extensor.

- Cortical myoclonus is frequently multifocal rather than focal.

  - Epilepsia partialis continua is repetitive focal cortical myoclonus with some rhythmicity.[2]

  - Any type of focal cortical lesion, including tumors, angiomas, and encephalitis, may be associated with focal cortical myoclonus. Rarely, Huntington's disease may cause cortical myoclonus.[3,4]

  - Epilepsia partialis continua can occur in focal encephalitis as in Rasmussen's syndrome,[5] in stroke, in tumors, and, rarely, in multiple sclerosis.[6]

- Sometimes, the cortex may be normal, and the responsible lesion is in the subcortical region.

  - Reflex myoclonus may be seen in Parkinson's disease (PD),[7] multiple systems atrophy, and cortical-basal ganglionic degeneration.[8]

  - In PD, it usually occurs distally and bilaterally, affecting the patient's wrist and fingers. It is characteristically an action myoclonus, irregular, small-amplitude, and multidirectional, at an average frequency of one jerk every 1–5 seconds. No relation to levodopa dose or motor severity has been found.[9]

  - Reflex myoclonus has also been reported to occur in Rett's syndrome and in Angelman's syndrome.[10,11]

- In children, myoclonus is usually associated with epilepsy. The major syndromes include infantile spasms and Lennox-Gastaut syndrome.[12] It is important to distinguish infantile spasms from benign myoclonus of infancy in which the electroencephalogram (EEG) is normal and the course is nonprogressive.[13]

Brainstem Myoclonus

There are three general types classified under brainstem myoclonus—exaggerated startle syndrome (hyperekplexia), brainstem reticular myoclonus (generalized muscle jerks), palatal myoclonus.

- Startle syndromes are characterized by an exaggerated startle response to a surprise stimulus. The normal startle response consists of blink and activation of other craniocervical muscles with a latency between the stimulus and electromyographic (EMG) activity of 30 seconds to 40 seconds.[14] Normal persons habituate quickly.

  - Hyperekplexia is a familial condition with symptoms starting in infancy.

  - Enhanced startle occurs in response to any type of stimulus, with generalized stiffening and falling to the ground.

  - The EMG latency is shorter than the normal startle response, and burst duration is brief.[15]

- Palatal myoclonus (sometimes called palatal tremor) is usually rhythmic. Because of its rhythmicity, the movements may resemble tremor; however, they have a jerky component, justifying usage of the term *myoclonus*.

  - Palatal myoclonus is usually continuous, independent of rest, action, sleep, or distraction.

  - It may occur unilaterally or bilaterally and results in 1.5- to 3-Hz movements that may also involve other muscles, including those of the eye, tongue, neck, and diaphragm.[16]

  - Palatal myoclonus may be due to a variety of neurologic disorders such as stroke, encephalitis, tumors, multiple sclerosis, trauma, and neurodegenerative disorders,[17] or it may be idiopathic.[18]

  - There may be an associated rhythmic clicking noise that is more likely to occur in cases of essential palatal myoclonus as compared to symptomatic palatal myoclonus.[18]

- Familial nocturnal faciomandibular myoclonus is a rare condition characterized by myoclonus involving the masseters and, subsequently, the orbicularis oris and oculi, resembling brainstem reticular myoclonus. It usually occurs during stage 2 of nonrapid eye movement sleep, and can result in tongue biting and bleeding.[19]

Spinal Myoclonus

Two forms of spinal myoclonus are now recognized: (1) spinal segmental myoclonus, affecting a restricted body part, involving a few spinal segments; and (2) propriospinal myoclonus, producing generalized axial jerks, usually beginning in the abdominal muscles.[20] Peripheral myoclonus is rare and can be seen with lesions of the nerve,[21] plexus,[22] or root.[17]

- Spinal myoclonus is associated with inflammatory myelopathy,[23] cervical spondylosis, tumors,[24] trauma,[25] ischemic myelopathy,[26] and a variety of other causes.[17] Occasionally, there is no identifiable cause.

- The possible mechanisms in "primary" spinal myoclonus include loss of inhibitory function, abnormal hyperactivity of local dorsal horn interneurons, aberrant local axon reexcitation, and loss of inhibition from suprasegmental descending pathways.[27]

Peripheral Myoclonus

Peripheral myoclonus has been described in lesions of the peripheral nerve, plexus, and root. The "ephaptic" transmission of peripheral ectopically generated potentials has been a proposed mechanism.[28]

Multifocal and Generalized Myoclonus

Multifocal myoclonus is characterized by individual jerks affecting different parts of the body. In generalized myoclonus, each jerk affects a large area or the entire body. Either form can be stimulus sensitive. Minipolymyoclonus is a form of multifocal myoclonus and is characterized by small jerks in different locations.[29] This term has also been used to describe small-amplitude jerks in patients with spinal muscular atrophy. The distinction can be made by the company these jerks keep (i.e., evidence of denervation in spinal muscular atrophy). Another variant of cortical reflex myoclonus is cortical tremor, which results in fine, shivering finger twitching provoked mainly by action and posture phenomenologically similar to essential tremor.[30] Cortical tremor may be familial.[31]

- Multifocal myoclonus is frequently due to metabolic causes including hepatic failure, uremia, hyponatremia, hypoglycemia, and nonketotic hyperglycemia. Toxic encephalopathies causing myoclonus include bismuth, methyl bromide, and toxic cooking oil.[32]

  - Lance-Adams syndrome refers to action myoclonus occurring after hypoxic brain injury with associated asterixis, seizures, and gait problems.[33] It is a multifocal myoclonus that improves with time and is rarely associated with severe additional neurologic deficits.

- Generalized myoclonus may be triggered by external stimuli and aggravated by action. In reticular reflex myoclonus, the origin of electrical discharge is usually in the brainstem. In this type of myoclonus, proximal muscles are more affected than distal ones and flexors are more active than extensors.[34]

  - The etiologies include spinocerebellar degenerations, mitochondrial disease (myoclonus epilepsy with ragged-red fibers), storage diseases (e.g., GM2 gangliosidoses), ceroid lipofuscinosis, sialidosis, and dementias such as Creutzfeldt-Jakob disease and Alzheimer's disease.

  - Viral and postviral syndromes may cause myoclonus.

Progressive Myoclonic Epilepsy

Progressive myoclonic epilepsies are a heterogeneous group of disorders associated with multifocal or generalized myoclonus and epileptic seizures. Under this category, two major groups exist: (1) the progressive myoclonic epilepsies (Figure 3.2) and (2) the progressive myoclonic ataxias.

- Progressive myoclonic epilepsies are a combination of severe myoclonus, generalized tonic-clonic, or other seizures and progressive neurologic decline, particularly dementia and ataxia. In the young, the following five conditions may cause progressive myoclonic epilepsy:

1. Lafora body disease is characterized by polyglucosan–Schiff-positive inclusion bodies in the brain, liver, muscle, or skin (eccrine sweat gland).

2. Neuronal ceroid lipofuscinosis (Batten's disease) presents with seizures, myoclonus, and dementia, along with blindness (in the childhood forms), and is characterized by curvilinear inclusion bodies in the brain, eccrine glands, muscle, and gut.

3. Unverricht-Lundborg disease is characterized by stimulus-sensitive myoclonus, tonic-clonic seizures, a characteristic EEG (paroxysmal generalized spike-wave activity and photosensitivity), ataxia, and mild dementia with an onset at around 5 to 15 years of age.

4. Myoclonic epilepsy with ragged-red fibers is maternally inherited, diagnosed by increased serum and cerebrospinal fluid (CSF) lactate and ragged-red fibers on muscle biopsy.

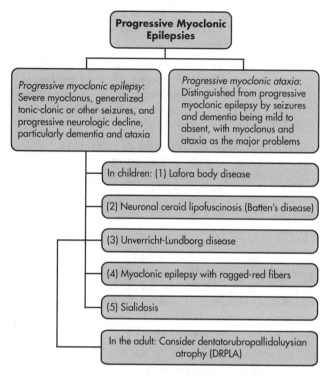

FIGURE 3.2
Classification of progressive myoclonic epilepsies.

5. Sialidosis is a lysosomal storage disorder associated with a cherry-red spot by funduscopy and dysmorphic facial features.

■ In the adult, dentatorubropallidoluysian atrophy is a consideration. It is more often seen in Japanese patients but has been described in other countries as well.[35,36] In the United States, it is most often described among African Americans in the Southeast (Haw River syndrome).

Progressive Myoclonic Ataxia (Ramsay Hunt Syndrome)

Progressive myoclonic ataxia (also known as Ramsay Hunt syndrome) is distinguished from progressive myoclonic epilepsy by seizures and dementia that are mild to absent, with myoclonus and ataxia as the major problems. It has a much wider span of presentation, ranging from the first to the seventh decade. The syndrome may be due either to recognizable etiology or to neurodegenerative disease.

- Known causes include mitochondrial encephalomyopathy, celiac disease, late- onset neuronal ceroid lipofuscinosis, biotin-responsive encephalopathy, adult Gaucher's disease, action myoclonus renal failure syndrome, May-White syndrome, and Ekbom's syndrome.

- Neurodegenerative diseases including pure spinocerebellar degeneration, spinocerebellar plus dentatorubral degeneration, olivopontocerebellar atrophy, or dentatorubropallidoluysian atrophy may manifest as progressive myoclonic ataxia.

Asterixis

Asterixis results in lapses of maintained postures and is considered a form of negative myoclonus. It usually occurs in conjunction with multifocal myoclonus. This usually occurs with multifocal myoclonus in the setting of a metabolic encephalopathy and is generalized. Focal asterixis may also be seen in lesions of the thalamus, the putamen, and the parietal lobe.

Opsoclonus-Myoclonus Syndrome

Opsoclonus-myoclonus syndrome results in random chaotic saccadic eye movements in association with multifocal and generalized myoclonus.[37.]

- Opsoclonus-myoclonus in adults is idiopathic in about 50% of cases. Idiopathic opsoclonus-myoclonus occurs in younger patients, and the clinical evolution is more benign.

- The second most common cause is paraneoplastic, usually from ovarian cancer, melanoma, renal cell carcinoma,[38] and lymphoma.

- It has been associated with viral infections such as Epstein-Barr virus.[39]

- Neuroblastoma is a major consideration in children, mainly in tumors with diffuse and extensive lymphocytic infiltration and lymphoid follicles.

- Other causes include drugs, toxins, and nonketotic hyperglycemia.

Physiologic Myoclonus

In physiologic myoclonus, muscle jerks occur in certain circumstances in normal subjects such as sleep jerks and hiccups.

Psychogenic Myoclonus

Psychogenic myoclonus is a "voluntary" or "simulated" myoclonus. Jerks are usually stimulus evoked, are of variable latency, and are usually longer than a voluntary reaction time.

Myoclonus-Dystonia Syndrome

Myoclonus-dystonia syndrome is a genetically heterogeneous autosomal dominant disorder with reduced penetrance and variable expression.[40] It is usually characterized by proximal bilateral myoclonic jerks, mainly involving the arms and axial muscles. A mild dystonia often presents as cervical dystonia or writer's cramp. The myoclonus can be rhythmic or arrhythmic, action provoked, and asymmetrical, and may or may not be alcohol responsive. Various combinations of myoclonus and dystonia in members of the same family have been seen. The variability of phenotypes suggests allelic mutations of the same gene.[40] The onset is usually in the first or second decade of life, both sexes are equally affected, and the course is relatively benign with a normal life span. Dementia, ataxia, and seizures are absent.

Drugs

Drugs that induce myoclonus include anticonvulsants, levodopa, lithium, and monoamine oxidase inhibitors. Lithium has been described to cause multifocal action myoclonus of cortical origin without epileptiform abnormalities on routine EEG. Fentanyl may cause myoclonus. Propofol has been reported to cause transient cortical reflex myoclonus that requires no treatment. Tricyclic antidepressants may cause an encephalopathy and myoclonus with EEG changes that may be confused with Creutzfeldt-Jakob disease. Mefloquine, used in chloroquine-resistant *Plasmodium falciparum* malaria, caused multifocal myoclonus in one patient. Amantadine has been reported to cause cortical myoclonus with EEG changes. Tardive myoclonus has been described following exposure to long-term neuroleptics. Newer antiepileptic drugs such as lamotrigine, gabapentin, and carvedilol (a beta blocker) and antibiotics such as gatifloxacin have been reported to induce myoclonus.

GENETICS

- Progressive myoclonic epilepsy, Lafora body disease, neuronal ceroid lipofuscinosis, Unverricht-Lundborg disease, and sialidosis are all autosomal recessive, whereas myoclonic epilepsy with ragged-red fibers is maternally inherited.

  - In Unverricht-Lundborg disease, the gene has now been localized to the long arm of chromosome 21q 22.3 in Finnish and Mediterranean families. The underlying gene encodes cystatin B, a cysteine protease inhibitor.[41] The major mutation worldwide is an unstable expansion of a dodecamer minisatellite repeat unit in the promoter region of the cystatin B gene. In addition, five "minor" mutations have been described.[42]

  - The gene for Lafora progressive myoclonic epilepsy maps to chromosome 6q23-25. It is caused by mutations in exon 1 of the EPM2A gene, which codes for laforin, a protein of unknown function.[43]

  - Sialidosis has been shown to be caused by mutations in the sialidase gene.

  - A variety of mutations have been described in myoclonic epilepsy–ragged-red fibers syndrome. It is typically associated with point mutations in the mtDNA tRNALys gene; however, double mutations may be seen.[44] In multiple symmetrical lipomatosis, myoclonus, and ataxia, mitochondrial DNA mutations may be seen.

  - Severe myoclonic epilepsy in infancy is characterized by normal development before onset, seizures beginning during first year of life in the form of generalized or unilateral febrile clonic seizures, and secondary appearance of myoclonic and partial seizures. This condition is refractory to medical treatment and is associated with ataxia and mental decline. There have been identified nonsense and frameshift mutations in the neuronal voltage-gated sodium channel alpha-subunit type I gene.[45]

- Dentatorubropallidoluysian atrophy is known as one of the CAG repeat expansion diseases in which the responsible gene is located on chromosome 12p and its product is called atrophin 1.[46] Dentatorubropallidoluysian atrophy shows prominent "anticipation," which is explained by a marked instability of the expanded CAG repeat length during spermatogenesis.

- The candidate region for myoclonus-dystonia is the chromosome 7q21-q31. It is inherited as an autosomal dominant trait with incomplete penetrance that appears to occur predominantly if the disease allele is passed on by the mother, suggesting maternal imprinting (i.e., differences in expression are dependent primarily on the sex of the transmitting parent). The gene for tachykinin 1, the precursor for substance P, is located in this region. Different heterozygous, loss-of-function mutations in the gene for epsilon-sarcoglycan are highly expressed in the central nervous system (CNS), and play a role in the dystrophin-glycoprotein complex. These areas have been identified and seem to play a role in this syndrome,[47] but additional genetic heterogeneity is suspected based on several spontaneous and familial cases without mutations in this gene. A missense mutation in the third exon of the gene for the dopamine (D2) receptor on chromosome 11q was found in one family.[48] However, this alteration has not been discovered in other families. Also, a novel gene related to myoclonus-dystonia was found on chromosome 18p11.[49]

- Hereditary hyperreflexia, transmitted as an autosomal dominant trait, has been linked to chromosome 5q33-q35, and the abnormal gene has now been identified to a point mutation in the alpha-1 subunit of the glycine receptor.

- Recently, the gene for familial adult myoclonic epilepsy (an autosomal dominant adult-onset condition characterized by "cortical tremor," various degrees of myoclonus in the limbs, and a benign course) has been localized to chromosome 8q24.[50] The cortical tremor is an action and postural finger tremor with electrophysiologic features of cortical reflex myoclonus. The same phenotype showed linkage to chromosome 2p11.1-q12.2, indicating that this disorder is a genetically heterogeneous condition.

- Finally, a new pedigree of a nonprogressive disorders with onset between the ages of 12 and 50 years (characterized by distal, semicontinuous rhythmic myoclonus, generalized tonic-clonic seizures, EEG abnormalities, and somatosensory and visual potentials of high amplitude) has been localized in the centromeric region of chromosome 2. The pattern of inheritance is autosomal dominant with high penetrance.[51]

DIFFERENTIAL DIAGNOSIS

The differential diagnosis of an isolated myoclonic jerk includes chorea and tic.

- Isolated choreic jerk may be indistinguishable from myoclonus; however, choreic jerk is not stimulus sensitive and tends to be not as rapid as myoclonus. In its fully developed form, chorea results in continuous random, flowing, quick, arrhythmic movements. Further, motor impersistence occurs and may manifest as an inability to keep the tongue protruded and also as waxing and waning of the grip strength (milkmaid's grip).

- Tic is a movement that may be simple or complex. In contrast to myoclonus, tics may be preceded by premonitory sensations, and their execution may be delayed or suppressed. Voluntary suppression of tics results in a build-up of inner tension that is relieved by the execution of the movement. In Tourette's syndrome, multiple motor and vocal tics may be associated with coprolalia and obsessive-compulsive symptoms.

- Dystonic movements can be rapid and may be confused with myoclonus. The term *myoclonic dystonia* refers to a combination of myoclonus and dystonia in other muscles. Sometimes, myoclonic dystonia is familial and may respond to alcohol.

- Terminal kinetic tremor and cerebellar ataxia may be severe enough to be confused with myoclonus. The two may coexist as in progressive myoclonic ataxia, and only after the treatment of myoclonus can the true severity of the underlying ataxia be appreciated.

- Some patients with postural tremor may have changes in amplitude, giving the impression of myoclonus, but rarely do these two conditions coexist.

DIAGNOSTIC WORKUP

The initial step is to identify the type of myoclonus. Clinical features may help, but sophisticated neurophysiologic testing may be necessary. These include EMG to determine the sequence of contractions, measurement of EMG burst duration, jerk-locked back-averaging, measurement of C reflexes to look for reflex production of myoclonus, and somatosensory evoked responses to look for giant somatosensory evoked potentials.

TABLE 3.1
Diagnostic Workup of a Patient with Myoclonus

Test	Purpose
EEG*	Rule out myoclonic epilepsy
MRI	Look for focal lesions
SPECT scan	To determine hyperexcitable region in cortical myoclonus
Cerebrospinal fluid	If infection is suspected
Metabolic workup: liver and kidney function, blood gases, blood sugar	For generalized or multifocal myoclonus if metabolic etiology is suspected
Visual evoked response and ERG	If neuronal ceroid lipofuscinosis is suspected
White cell or fibroblast lysosomal enzyme estimations	To rule out sialidosis or other lysosomal storage disorders
Screening for urinary oligosaccharides and organic acids	If progressive myoclonic epilepsies are suspected
Plasma and cerebrospinal fluid lactate	If mitochondrial encephalopathy is suspected
Skin and conjunctival biopsy and electromicroscopy	To rule out neuronal ceroid lipofuscinosis, Lafora body disease, and neuroaxonal dystrophy
Muscle biopsy	To look for ragged-red fibers and to study mitochondrial metabolism
Jejunal biopsy	To look for celiac disease and Whipple's disease
Anti-Ri antibodies may be positive in the DRPLA gene test	For opsoclonus-myoclonus syndrome. For adult-onset progressive myoclonic epilepsy.

*Back-averaging EEGs represents the best available test for physiologically proving myoclonus.

The type of myoclonus and associated features guide further workup (Table 3.1).

- Routine surface EEG may fail to show spikes in cortical reflex myoclonus and may be normal in epilepsia partialis continua.

- Electrocorticography may be needed to find the abnormal discharge.

- An imaging study, preferably an MRI (magnetic resonance imaging) study, should be performed to look for focal lesions.

- A single photon emission computed tomography (SPECT) activation study can be employed to determine the hyperexcitable region in cortical myoclonus.[52]

- The cerebrospinal fluid should be examined if infection is suspected.

- In generalized and multifocal myoclonus, the metabolic workup should include testing for liver and kidney functions, blood gases, and measurement of blood sugar.

- In patients with progressive myoclonic epilepsy and progressive myoclonic ataxia:

    - The diagnostic workup should include visual evoked responses and EEG to rule out seizures in neuronal ceroid lipofuscinosis.

    - Elevated plasma and cerebrospinal fluid lactate point to a mitochondrial encephalomyopathy.

    - White cell or fibroblast lysosomal enzyme estimations are necessary, as is screening for urinary oligosaccharides and organic acids.

    - Skin and conjunctival biopsy and electromicroscopy (to look for inclusions in nerves, especially in eccrine sweat glands, in neuronal ceroid lipofuscinosis, Lafora body disease, and neuroaxonal dystrophy), muscle biopsy (to look for ragged-red fibers and to study mitochondrial metabolism), and jejunal biopsy (to look for celiac disease and Whipple's disease).

- Anti-Ri antibodies may be positive in the opsoclonus-myoclonus syndrome.

- Palatal myoclonus needs to be investigated by an MRI to look for lesions in the Guillain-Mollaret triangle. In many cases, olivary hypertrophy may be appreciable on MRI by a change in signal in the olive. The type and location of the lesion (i.e., stroke versus multiple plaques) will guide further workup.

- In spinal myoclonus, appropriate imaging studies and examination of cerebrospinal fluid is indicated.

TREATMENT

The most important initial step is to try to subclassify the type of myoclonus and to identify the underlying disease process.

- Metabolic derangements or other underlying conditions, if found, need to be treated.

TABLE 3.2
Management of Myoclonus

Condition/indication	Treatment
First-line treatment for the symptomatic control of myoclonus	Clonazepam (4–10 mg per day) Sodium valproate (250–4500 mg per day) Piracetam (10–24 g per day)
Other options for symptomatic treatment of myoclonus	Lisuride Acetazolamide Carbamazepine Leviteracetam Neurontin
Lance-Adams or postanoxic myoclonus	Combination of 5-hydroxytryptophan (600–2000 mg per day) and carbidopa (100–200 mg per day)
Palatal myoclonus	Often resistant to therapy; may try anticholinergics; 5-hydroxytryptophan; carbamazepine
Myoclonus-dystonia syndrome and severe treatment-refractory myoclonus	Consider deep brain stimulation
Essential myoclonus	Try anticholinergics
Spinal myoclonus	Surgical removal of etiology; may try clonazepam or tetrabenazine

- A number of different drugs have been used for the symptomatic control of myoclonus (Table 3.2).

  - The most effective drugs are clonazepam (4–10 mg per day), sodium valproate (250–4500 mg per day), and piracetam (10–24 g per day).

  - Somewhat less effective drugs include lisuride, acetazolamide, and carbamazepine.

  - In Lance-Adams syndrome and in posttraumatic action myoclonus, a combination of 5-hydroxytryptophan (600–2000 mg per day) and carbidopa (100–200 mg per day) can be effective. Adding two or three drugs in combination is often helpful for post-hypoxic myoclonus.

  - Recently, levetiracetam has been reported to alleviate posthypoxic, spinal, and postencephalitic myoclonus.

  - Several of these drugs can be used in combination to obtain a response, especially in cortical reflex myoclonus.

- Gabapentin was effective in myoclonus induced by chronic opiate medication in cancer patients with pain.

- Progressive myoclonic epilepsy may be worsened by phenytoin. Acetazolamide may be helpful in myoclonus of Ramsay Hunt syndrome.

- Essential myoclonus often responds to alcohol and may be improved by anticholinergics.

- Palatal myoclonus is usually resistant to therapy, but in some cases, anticholinergics, 5-hydroxytryptophan, and carbamazepine have been helpful.

- Spinal myoclonus may respond to removal of compressing lesion and effective drugs have included clonazepam and tetrabenazine.[17]

- Negative myoclonus often resolves with the correction of the responsible metabolic derangement, and ethosuximide may be particularly useful in the symptomatic treatment.

- One report describes a significant reduction of myoclonus and dystonic spasms in a case of myoclonus dystonia syndrome using oral gamma-hydroxybutyric acid, a drug used in the treatment of alcohol withdrawal.[53]

  - In addition, one patient with myoclonus-dystonia syndrome improved approximately 80% with neurostimulation of the ventralis intermedius thalamic nucleus without any significant change in the dystonic symptoms.[54]

  - Finally, another patient showed significant improvement in myoclonus and dystonia after medial pallidum stimulation.[55]

The prognosis depends on the underlying disorder causing myoclonus. No complications are related to isolated myoclonic jerks, but accompanying seizures may lead to hypoxia, injuries, and aspiration.

REFERENCES

1. Caviness J, Alving L, Maraganore D, et al. The incidence and prevalence of myoclonus in Olmsted County, Minnesota. Mayo Clin Proc 1999;74(6):565–569.
2. Hallett M. Early history of myoclonus. In: Fahn S, Marsden CD, Van Woert MH, eds. Advances in Neurology: Myoclonus. New York: Raven Press, 1986;43:7–10.
3. Thompson PD, Bhatia KP, Brown P, et al. Cortical myoclonus in Huntington's disease. Mov Disord 1994;9(6):633–641.

4. Caviness JN, Kurth M. Cortical myoclonus in Huntington's disease associated with an enlarged somatosensory evoked potential. Mov Disord 1997;12(6):1046–1051.

5. Cockerell OC, Rothwell J, Thompson PD, et al. Clinical and physiological features of epilepsia partialis continua. Cases ascertained in the UK. Brain 1996;119(Pt 2):393–407.

6. Hess DC, Sethi KD. Epilepsia partialis continua in multiple sclerosis. Int J Neurosci 1990;50:109–111.

7. Caviness JN, Adler CH, Newman S, et al. Cortical myoclonus in levodopa-responsive parkinsonism. Mov Disord 1998;13(3): 540–544.

8. Chen R, Ashby P, Lang AE. Stimulus-sensitive myoclonus in akinetic rigid syndromes. Brain 1992;115:1875–1888.

9. Caviness JN, Adler CH, Beach TG, et al. Small-amplitude cortical myoclonus in Parkinson's disease: physiology and clinical observations. Mov Disord 2002;17(4):657–662.

10. Guerrini R, Bonanni P, Parmeggiani L, et al. Cortical reflex myoclonus in Rett syndrome. Ann Neurol 1998;43(4):472–479.

11. Guerrini R, De Lorey TM, Bonanni P, et al. Cortical myoclonus in Angelman syndrome. Ann Neurol 1996;40(1):39–48.

12. Aicardi J. Myoclonic epilepsies of infancy and childhood. In: Fahn S, Marsden CD, Van Woert M, eds. Advances in Neurology: Myoclonus. New York: Raven Press, 1986;43:11–31.

13. Lombroso CT, Fejerman N. Benign myoclonus of early infancy. Ann Neurol 1977;1:38–43.

14. Wilkins DE, Hallett M, Wess MM. The audiogenic startle reflex of man and its relationship to startle syndromes. Brain 1986;109: 561–573.

15. Day BL, Marsden CD. The hyperrexplexias and their relationship to the normal startle reflex. Brain 1991;114:1903–1928.

16. Lapresle J. Palatal myoclonus. In: Fahn S, Marsden CD, Van Woert M, eds. Advances in Neurology: Myoclonus. New York: Raven Press, 1986;43:265–273.

17. Jankovic J, Pardo R. Segmental myoclonus: clinical and pharmacologic study. Arch Neurol 1986;43:1025–1031.

18. Deuschl G, Mischke G, Schenck E, et al. Symptomatic and essential rhythmic palatal myoclonus. Brain 1990;113:1645–1672.

19. Vetrugno R, Provini F, Plazzi G, et al. Familial nocturnal facio-mandibular myoclonus mimicking sleep bruxism. Neurology 2002;58(4):644–647.

20. Chokroverty S, Manocha MK, Duvoisin RC. A physiologic and pharmacologic study in anticholinergic-responsive essential myoclonus. Neurology 1987;37:608–615.

21. Marsden CD, Obeso JA, Traub MM, et al. Muscle spasm associated with Sudeck's atrophy after injury. Br Med J (Clin Res Ed) 1984;288:173–176.

22. Banks G, Nielsen VK, Short MP, Kowal CD. Brachial plexus myoclonus. J Neurol Neurosurg Psychiatry 1985;48:582–584.

23. Campbell AM, Garland H. Subacute myoclonic spinal neuronitis. J Neurol Neurosurg Psychiatry 1956;19:268–274.

24. Garcin R, Rondot P, Guiot G. Rhythmic myoclonus of the right arm as the presenting symptom of a cervical cord tumour. Brain 1968;91:75–84.

25. Brown P, Thompson PD, Rothwell JC, Day BL. Axial myoclonus of propriospinal origin. Brain 1991;114:197–214.

26. Davis SM, Murray NM, Diengdoh JV, et al. Stimulus-sensitive spinal myoclonus. J Neurol Neurosurg Psychiatry 1981;44:884–888.

27. Campos CR, Limongi JC, Machado FC, Brotto MW. A case of primary spinal myoclonus: clinical presentation and possible mechanisms involved. Arq Neuropsiquiatr 2003;61(1):112–114.

28. Martinez MS, Fontoira M, Celester G, et al. Myoclonus of peripheral origin : Case secondary to a digital nerve lesion. Mov Disord 2001;16(5):970–974.

29. Wilkins DE, Hallett M, Erba G. Primary generalized epileptic myoclonus: a frequent manifestation of minipolymyoclonus of central origin. J Neurol Neurosurg Psychiatry 1985;48:506–516.

30. Ikeda A, Kakigi R, Funai N, et al. Cortical tremor: a variant of cortical reflex myoclonus. Neurology 1990;40(10):1561–1565.

31. Elia M, Musumeci S, Ferri R, et al. Familial cortical tremor, epilepsy, and mental retardation: a distinct clinical entity? Arch Neurol 1998;55(12):1569–1573.

32. Obeso JA, Artieda J, Marsden CD. Different clinical presentations of myoclonus. In: Jankovic J, Tolosa E, eds. Parkinson's Disease and Movement Disorders. 2nd ed. Baltimore: Williams & Wilkins, 1993:315–328.

33. Lance JW, Adams RD. The syndrome of intention or action myoclonus as a sequel to hypoxic encephalopathy. Brain 1963;86:111–136.

34. Hallett M, Chadwick D, Adam J, Marsden CD. Reticular reflex myoclonus: a physiological type of human post-hypoxic myoclonus. J Neurol Neurosurg Psychiatry 1977b;40:253–264.

35. Naito H, Oyanagi S. Familial myoclonus epilepsy and choreoathetosis: hereditary dentatorubral-pallidoluysian atrophy. Neurology 1982;32:798–807.

36. Becher MW, Rubinsztein DC, Leggo J, et al. Dentatorubral and pallidoluysian atrophy (DRPLA). Clinical and neuropathological findings in genetically confirmed North American and European pedigrees. Mov Disord 1997;12(4):519–530.

37. Caviness JN, Forsyth PA, Layton DD, McPhee TJ. The movement disorder of adult opsoclonus. Mov Disord 1995;10(1):22–27.

38. Vigliani MC, Palmucci L, Polo P, et al. Paraneoplastic opsoclonus-myoclonus associated with renal cell carcinoma and responsive to tumor ablation. J Neurol Neurosurg Psychiatry 2001;70(6):814–815.

39. Verma A, Brozman B. Opsoclonus-myoclonus syndrome following Epstein-Barr virus infection. Neurology 2002;58:1131–1132.

40. Vidailhet M, Tassin J, Durif F, et al. A major locus for several phenotypes of myoclonus—dystonia on chromosome 7q. Neurology 2001;59:1213–1216.

41. Pennacchio LA, Lehesjoki AE, Stone NE, et al. Mutations in the gene encoding cystatin B in progressive myoclonus epilepsy (EPM1). Science 1996;271(5256):1731–1734.

42. Lehesjoki AE, Koskiniemi M. Progressive myoclonus epilepsy of Unverricht-Lundborg type. Epilepsia 1999;3(40 Suppl):23–28.

43. Minassian BA, Ianzano L, Meloche M, et al. Mutations spectrum and predicted function of laforin in Lafora's progressive myoclonus epilepsy. Neurology 2000;55(3):341–346.

44. Arenas J, Campos Y, Bornstein B, et al. A double mutation (A8296G and G8363A) in the mitochondrial DNA tRNA (Lys) gene associated with myoclonus epilepsy with ragged-red fibers. Neurology 1999;52(2):377–382.

45. Sugawara T, Mazaki-Miyazaki E, Fukushima K, et al. Frequent mutations of SCN1A in severe myoclonic epilepsy in infancy. Neurology 2002;58(7):1122–1124

46. Kanazawa I. Molecular pathology of dentatorubral-pallidoluysian atrophy. Philos Trans R Soc Lond B Biol Sci 1999;354(1386):1069–1074.

47. Zimprich A, Grabowski M, Asmus F, et al. Mutations in the gene encoding epsilon-sarcoglycan cause myoclonus-dystonia syndrome. Nat Genet 2001;29(1):66–69.

48. Klein C, Gurvich N, Sena-Esteves M, et al. Evaluation of the role of the D2 dopmaine receptor in myoclonus dystonia. Ann Neurol 2000;47(3):369–373.

49. Grimes DA, Han F, Lang AE, et al. A novel locus for inherited myoclonus-dystonia on 18p11. Neurology 2002;59(8):1187–1196.

50. Plaster NM, Uyama E, Uchino M, et al. Genetic localization of the familial adult-myoclonic epilepsy (FAME) gene to chromosome 8q24. Neurology 1999;53(6):1180–1183.

51. Guerrini R, Bonanni P, Patrignani A, et al. Autosomal dominant cortical myoclonus and epilepsy (ADCME) with complex partial and generalized seizures: a newly recognized epilepsy syndrome with linkage to chromosome 2p11.1-q12.2. Brain 2001;124(Pt 12):2459–2475.

52. Tanaka K, Suga R, Yamada T, et al. Idiopathic cortical myoclonus restricted to the lower limbs: correlation between MEPs and 99mTc-ECD single photon emission computed tomography activation study. J Neurol Sci 1999;163(1):58–60.

53. Priori A, Berolasi L, Pesenti A. Gamma-hydroxybutyric acid for alcohol sensitive myoclonus with dystonia. Neurology 2000;54:1706.

54. Kupsch A. Neurostimulation of the ventral intermediate thalamic nucleus in inherited myoclonus-dystonia syndrome. Mov Disord 2001;16(4):769–771.

55. Liu X, Griffin I, Parkin S, et al. Involvement of the medial pallidum in focal myoclonic dystonia: a clinical and neurophysiological case study. Mov Disord 2002;17(2):346–353.

4

THE "SHAKY" PATIENT

PHENOMENOLOGY

Tremors are involuntary, regular, rhythmic, oscillatory, to-and-fro movements of a body part or region that results from the alternating contraction of opposing muscles.

- Tremors may affect any body region, but more commonly affects hands and fingers, followed by the tongue, head, jaw, legs, and trunk.

- Tremors may occur in isolation but frequently they are associated with clinical syndromes.

- Careful evaluation of the tremor characteristics is essential for classification and diagnosis and includes careful observation of the frequency, amplitude, rhythm, and triggering conditions.

CLASSIFICATION (Table 4.1)

Resting tremors (RT) occur when the extremity is in complete repose and subside with activation or movement of the affected body part.

Postural tremors occur when the affected limb is held against gravity or in a particular position.

Action or *kinetic tremors* occur when the affected limb is involved in any particular movement.

TABLE 4.1
Syndromic Classification of Common Tremor Disorders

Type	Characteristic	Tremor Frequency (Hz)
Parkinsonian tremor	Rest >> posture = action	3–6
Enhanced physiologic tremor	Action = posture	8–12
Essential tremor	Action > posture >> rest	4–10
Cerebellar tremor	Action	2–4
Rubral tremor	Posture = action > rest	2–5
Orthostatic tremor	Only when standing still; relieved by walking or sitting	15–18
Dystonic tremor	Posture = action >> rest	4–8
Palatal tremor	Rest	1–6
Neuropathic tremor	Posture >> action	5–9

Intention tremors occur during the performance of a projected movement with worsening of the amplitude with movement toward the target.

CLINICAL DISORDERS (Table 4.2)

Enhanced Physiologic Tremor

Enhanced physiologic tremor (EPT) is, for the most part, a high-frequency postural tremor that is not the result of neurologic illness but may be a result of metabolic or toxic disorders.

- Trigger conditions include hyperthyroidism, liver disease, benzodiazepine withdrawal, lithium, valproate, calcium channel blockers, anxiety, and hypoglycemia.

- Usually not a disabling tremor but mostly a cause of concern for patients who may think they are developing a neurodegenerative disorder.

Parkinson's Disease (see also Chapter 5)

The classic condition associated with resting tremor is Parkinson's disease (PD), but resting tremors may also be observed in other parkinsonian syndromes.

TABLE 4.2
Tremor Characteristics by Condition

Diagnosis	Predominant Tremor	Remarks
Parkinson's disease	Resting tremor	Associated symptoms include rigidity, bradykinesia, and postural instability. Usually an elderly patient (>50 y/o), with asymmetric onset, 4–6 Hz
Essential tremors	Postural tremors	Kinetic tremors may be appreciated, usually symmetric, responds to alcohol, bimodal age of onset (teens, >50 y/o), 4–10 Hz
Cerebellar tremors	Intention tremors	Postural component may be present, other ataxic features on exam. Seen with alcoholism and stroke, 2–4 Hz
Holmes' tremors	Rest, posture, and intention	Seen in multiple sclerosis and traumatic brain injury, 2–5 Hz
Dystonic tremor	Posture and intention	Abnormal posture of affected limb may be observed, variable frequency, 4–8 Hz
Enhanced physiologic tremors	Postural tremor	Check for metabolic disorders (thyroid, diabetes, renal failure, liver disease) or tremor-inducing drugs, 8–12 Hz
Orthostatic tremors	Postural, in the legs, upon standing	Usually occurs when patient stands up, improves with ambulation, 15–18 Hz
Palatal tremor	Postural	1–6 Hz
Neuropathic tremors	Posture, kinetic	In association with neuropathy, 5–9 Hz

- Because this tremor mostly occurs at rest, it is often not associated with significant functional disability but with social embarrassment.

- The characteristic frequency (not always this frequency) associated with this tremor is 4–6 Hz. It often starts intermittently, then gradually becomes persistent.

- The most common areas affected include the hands, legs, lips, and jaw. Patients frequently complain of the sensation of internal tremors that are not visible from the outside.

- In Parkinson's disease, postural and intention tremors (often of lesser severity) may be appreciated.

- The clue is the presence of associated symptoms in PD which include[1]: rigidity, bradykinesia, and postural instability.

  - A characteristic feature of symptoms in PD is the asymmetrical nature, especially early in the disease.

  - Other associated findings include masked facies, asymmetrical arm swing, stooped posture, difficulty turning, and hypophonia.

Essential Tremor

Essential tremor (ET) is the most common tremor syndrome seen in adults.

- The characteristic tremors seen in ET are postural and action tremors, with a frequency of 4 or greater Hz.

- Although frequently seen in the elderly (thus previously called "senile tremors"), ETs may begin insidiously early in life, with an increment in tremor severity over the years.

- Unlike PD, the disability in ET is associated with impairment of voluntary activities that occur as a result of the tremor.

  - Patients commonly complain of tremors when eating, drinking, and writing, spilling food and drinks and developing a progressively illegible handwriting.

- Most commonly affected body parts include hands, head, and voice, but tremors can also be seen in the legs, trunk, and face.

  - Despite being mainly a postural tremor and kinetic tremor, a resting tremor of lesser severity can sometimes be seen.

- The tremor in ET is exacerbated by conditions such as stress, exercise, fatigue, caffeine, and certain medications and the tremor improves with relaxation and alcohol.

- Several tremor conditions are believed to be variants of essential tremor including:

  - Task-specific tremor (e.g., primary writing tremor)

  - Isolated voice tremor

  - Isolated chin tremor

Cerebellar Tremor

Cerebellar tremor is a slow-frequency tremor, between 3 and 5 Hz. It occurs during the execution of a goal-directed movement (intentional).

- The amplitude frequently increases with the movement (usually by approaching the intended target) and can be associated with a postural component.

- Other findings suggestive of ataxia may be found on physical examination.

  - Another tremor associated with a cerebellar etiology is titubation, better described as a slow-frequency "bobbing" motion of the head or trunk.

  - It is usually seen in conditions as multiple sclerosis, hereditary ataxia syndromes, brainstem stroke affecting cerebellar pathways, and traumatic brain injury.

  - Unfortunately, these tremors are highly disabling and are very difficult to treat.

Holmes' Tremor

Holmes' tremor is believed to result from lesions affecting the cerebellothalamic and nigrostriatal pathways.

- Characterized by resting, postural, and intention tremors of a low frequency (<4.5 Hz), affecting the proximal limbs more than distal.

- Usually associated with central nervous system (CNS) lesions in the midbrain and superior cerebellar peduncles and thalamus and may be seen in patients with multiple sclerosis and traumatic brain injury.

- Associated with enormous disability and is commonly resistant to treatment.

Dystonic Tremor

As the name implies, dystonic tremor is a tremor that occurs in a body region affected by dystonia.

- Presents as a postural/action tremor with irregular amplitudes and frequencies.

- An example of this tremor is dystonic, no-no or yes-yes head tremor associated with spasmodic torticollis. This tremor tends to be irregular or arrhythmical and may improve with antagonistic gestures (geste antagoniste), in contrast to the rhythmical head tremor resulting from ET.

Neuropathic Tremor

Neuropathic tremors are mostly postural or action tremors that occur in the setting of a peripheral neuropathy.

- More commonly associated with demyelinating neuropathies of the dysgammaglobulinemic type.[2]

- Frequency often described between 3 and 6 Hz in hand and arm muscles.

- Exact etiology is unknown.

Palatal Tremor (see also Chapter 3)

Palatal tremors are classified in two forms: symptomatic and essential.

1. Symptomatic palatal tremor, secondary to brainstem/cerebellar lesions, results from rhythmic contraction of the tensor veli palatini. Movement of the edge of the palate is appreciated.

2. Essential palatal tremor is not associated with CNS lesions and is a result of rhythmic contractions of the tensor veli palatini, associated with an ear click. Movement of the roof of the palate is also seen.

Drug-Induced Tremors

Drug-induced tremors may be seen at rest, with posture or with intention, and the presentation is dependent on the offending agent. Drugs associated with tremor induction include, e.g., centrally acting agents (neuroleptics, antidepressants), sympathomimetics, steroids, immunosuppressive agents, bronchodilators, alcohol, caffeine, valproic acid, amiodarone, nicotine, and lithium (Table 4.3).

Hysterical Tremor

Also known as psychogenic tremor, hysterical tremor usually presents a challenge in any neurologic practice.

TABLE 4.3
List of Potential Toxins and Drugs Inducing Tremor[3-5]

Toxins	Drugs
Nicotine	Neuroleptics
Mercury	Reserpine
Lead	Tetrabenazine
Carbon monoxide	Metoclopramide
Manganese	Antidepressants
Arsenic	Lithium
Cyanide	Cocaine
Naphthalene	Adrenaline
Alcohol	Theophylline
Phosphorus	Caffeine
Toluene	Dopamine
DDT	Steroids
Lindane	Valproate
Kepone	Perhexiline
Dioxins	Antiarrhythmics (amiodarone)
Cytostatics (vincristine, adriablastin, cytosine arabinoside, ifosfamide)	Mexiletine, procainamide
Immunosuppressants (cyclosporine A)	Calcitonin
Thyroid hormones	

- Usually has an irregular frequency and is associated with sudden onset and remissions, frequency and amplitude may diminish or disappear with distraction, "coactivation sign" may be observed, and other somatization historical points may be appreciated.

Orthostatic Tremor

Orthostatic tremor is mostly confined to the legs (but has also been reported in the arms and jaw) and will occur upon standing and will subside with walking.

- There is no problem when sitting or lying down.

TABLE 4.4
Clinical Examination of the Tremulous Patient

Technique	Examination technique	Findings
Observe	What is the affected body region?	Assess the degree of disability, if head tremors only, consider spasmodic torticollis
	Is there an abnormal body posture?	Suggests a dystonic tremor
	Does the tremor occur at rest, or is it associated with purposeful movement?	Tremor at rest suggests PD Tremor with posture/intention suggests ET or other disorders.
	Are there leg tremors?	If the tremors occur only upon standing, orthostatic tremors is the most likely diagnosis; resting tremors while sitting is more suggestive of PD
	Is there masked facies?	The presence of masked facies or shuffling gait suggests parkinsonism
	Is there reduced amplitude of movement?	Assess with finger taps, patient open and close hand for 10 seconds, presence suggests parkinsonism
	Is there voice tremor?	Suggestive of ET and dystonia; also seen in other condition but less pronounced
	Is there shuffling gait?	Suggestive of parkinsonism
Examine	With the patient keeping the extremities at rest, distract patient by asking to perform serial sevens	This maneuver may provoke the emergence of resting tremors
	Examine extremities in postural position (hands in front of patient, parallel to floor)	Postural tremors suggests ET, if fast frequency, exaggerated physiologic tremors/neuropathic tremors/cerebellar tremors
	Finger to nose testing	If there is intention tremors and: • Ataxia, suggests cerebellar or Holmes tremors • Intention tremors on its own, ET dystonia, suggests dystonic tremors
	Examine for rigidity and bradykinesia; decreased arm swing	Presence of this suggests PD or any parkinsonian syndrome

TABLE 4.4 (cont.)

Technique	Examination technique	Findings
Stance/ gait	Examination of casual gait	• Shuffling suggests parkinsonian syndromes • Wide-based gait suggests the presence of ataxia • Freezing of gait suggests parkinsonian disorders • Abnormal body postures suggests dytonia
	Tandem gait	• Abnormalities may be seen in ataxia and ET
Speech evaluation	Prepared text may be helpful; e.g., "The Rainbow Passage" (see Appendix)	• Altered articulation of words • Abnormal fluency • Slowed speech • "Scanning dysarthria"—words are broken into syllables • Voice tremors

■ The tremor rate is between 13 and 18 Hz (via electromography [EMG])

■ Treatment includes clonazepam or primidone.

Physiologic Tremor

Physiologic tremor is a high-frequency, small-amplitude tremor that is seen in normal individuals. The usual for hand tremor is between 6 and 12 Hz

■ Enhanced physiologic tremor (EPT) is a visible predominantly as a postural, high-frequency tremor of short duration (<2 years).

■ Can be from endogenous or exogenous intoxication; aggravated by stress and hyperthyroidism

EVALUATION OF THE TREMULOUS PATIENT

Once the patient history is reviewed and history of neuropathy, drug use, toxic exposure, and family history of tremors is obtained, proceed with the physical examination (Table 4.4).

Diagnostic Workup (Table 4.5)

Treatment

TABLE 4.5 Diagnostic Workup for Tremors		
Thyroid function tests	If hypo-/hyperthyroid, treat as neccesary	Thyroid disorders, in particular hyperthyroidism, are associated with tremors
Liver function studies	Screen for liver disease	Hepatic encephalopathy may be associated with tremors
Complete chemistry	Correct metabolic disturbances as neccessary	Uremia may induce tremors
Serum ceruloplasmin	Usually obtained in patients <50 y/o	24-hr urine collection for copper excretion also recommended
Toxicology screen	Assess for drug-induced, illicit drug use, toxic etiology (e.g., mercury, lead)	Drug abuse/withdrawal, ethyl alcohol withdrawal may be associated with tremors, other signs may be present
Drug levels	Antiepileptic drugs, immunosuppressants	Cyclosporine, valproate
MRI of the brain	Assess for structural, demyelinating, vascular lesions	Cerebellar lesions for cerebellar tremors

Parkinson's Disease

The resting tremor in PD usually responds to dopaminergic therapy (dopamine agonists, levodopa) and anticholinergics (Table 4.6). Levodopa is the most efficacious medication, sometimes resulting in dramatic tremor suppression. It may be combined with dopamine agonists or anticholinergics in resistant patients. For patients with disabling tremors not responding to usual dosages, the dose should be escalated as tolerated. Side effects from medications are usually the limiting factor. For the patient who continues to have disabling, medication-refractory tremors after comprehensive medication trials or who cannot tolerate medications because of side effects, functional neurosurgery is an option.[6] The PD tremors have shown significant improvement with lesioning procedures or deep brain stimulation of the thalamus, globus pallidus, or subthalamic nucleus.[7, 8]

TABLE 4.6
Pharmacological Treatment Options for Newly Diagnosed
Parkinson's Disease*

Drug	Dose range	Comments
Carbidopa/levodopa	300–1200 mg/d	Nausea, vomiting, sedation, hallucinations
Ropinirole	3–24 mg/d	Nausea, vomiting, sedation, hallucinations, sleep attacks
Pramipexole	1.5–4.5 mg/d	Nausea, vomiting, sedation, hallucinations, sleep attacks
Pergolide	1–5 mg/d	Nausea, vomiting, sedation, hallucinations, cardiac valvular disease, sleep attacks
Trihexyphenidil	6–15 mg/d	Confusion, sedation, hallucinations, dry mouth, bladder retention
Benztropine	1–6 mg/d	Confusion, sedation, hallucinations, dry mouth, bladder retention
Amantadine	200–400 mg/d	Confusion, hallucinations, dry mouth, bladder retention, livido reticularis, leg edema
Selegiline	5 mg twice per day	Confusion, hallucinations
Rasagiline	0.5–1.0 mg/d	Confusion, hallucinations

*See also Chapter 5.

Essential Tremors

Propranolol and primidone are the preferred first-line treatments for ETs, alone or in combination (Table 4.7). There is often a better response for hand tremors, but these drugs are also recommended for head and voice tremors, although they seem to be less effective. The dose range for propranolol is from 10–240 mg divided three times a day, and for the long-acting formulation 60–320 mg, once or twice per day. The recommended dose range for primidone is 50–250 mg divided three times per day. Propranolol is contraindicated in patients suffering from asthma, diabetes, or cardiac arrhythmias. Primidone is associated with drowsiness, nausea, dizziness, and confusion. Gabapentin has also been shown to improve ET in two studies, with a dosage range of 1800–2400 mg divided three times per day. Topiramate, clonazepam, clozapine, and botulinum toxin have also been reported to

TABLE 4.7
Pharmacologic Therapy for Essential Tremors[9, 11]

Medication	Dosage*	Comments
Propranolol	10–240 mg divided bid-tid	Contraindicated in cardiac arrhythmias, diabetes, and pulmonary disorders. Watch for hypotension and depression
Propranolol LA (long-acting formulation)	60–320 mg qd-bid	Same as above
Primidone	50–750 mg divided tid or given qhs	Sedation, nausea, dizziness, confusion
Neurontin	900–2400 mg divided tid	Leucopenia, somnolence, dizziness, ataxia
Topiramate	Up to 400 mg/d	Paresthesias, anorexia, difficulty with concentration
Clonazepam	0.5–6 mg/d	Drowsiness

* Slow titration schedules recommended for all these medications to reduce incidence of side effects.

improve tremors in ET in multiple reports.[9] Patients experiencing worsening of tremors associated with anxiety may benefit from anxiolytics. For patients who continue to have disabling tremors despite optimal medical therapy and adequate medication trial or do not tolerate therapy as a result of side effects, thalamic lesioning or deep brain stimulation is an effective alternative.[10]

Cerebellar Tremors

No medication has shown consistent, successful treatment of cerebellar tremors. Medications that can be tried include clonazepam, propranolol, trihexyphenidil, levodopa, physostigmine, and topiramate.[12] Thalamic stimulation for disabling tremor may be an option, and referral to an experienced center may be helpful.[13]

Dystonic Tremors

Head, arm, and voice tremors resulting from dystonia have been shown to improve with botulinum toxin injections. Other medications that can be tried include anticholinergics, levodopa, propranolol, and clonazepam.[14]

Orthostatic Tremors

The treatment of choice for orthostatic tremors is low-dose clonazepam. Phenobarbital, primidone, propranolol, and neurontin may also be tried when clonazepam fails or is not tolerated.

Enhanced Physiologic Tremors

The most important step to treat EPTs is to discover the underlying cause. If a metabolic etiology is found during workup (e.g., thyroid, glucose), it should be treated accordingly. In the anxious patient, treatment of the anxiety may improve tremors. If drug induced, decrease the dosage or stop the offending drug.

Neuropathic Tremors

To date, there has been no successful pharmacologic treatment reported for the treatment of neuropathic tremors. Medications such as clonazepam, primidone, and propranolol have been tried with inconsistent benefit. A case of disabling neuropathic tremor has been reported to have benefited from thalamic deep brain stimulation, and this should be considered.[15]

Palatal Tremors

Palatal tremors are usually not disabling. Patients may be bothered by the ear click associated with EPT and may benefit from pharmacologic treatment with trihexyphenidil, valproate, and flunarizine. Injection of botulinum toxin in the tensor veli palatini has been reported to be beneficial.[16]

Drug-Induced Tremors

The treatment for drug-induced tremors usually consists of discontinuation or dose reduction of the offending agent.

REFERENCES

1. Tolosa E, Wenning G, Poewe W. The diagnosis of Parkinson's disease. Lancet Neurol 2006;5(1):75–86.
2. Bain PG, Britton TC, Jenkins IH, et al. Tremor associated with benign IgM paraproteinaemic neuropathy. Brain 1996;119 (Pt 3):789–799.

3. Karas BJ, Wilder BJ, Hammond EJ, Bauman AW. Valproate tremors. Neurology 1982;32(4):428–432.

4. LeDoux MS, McGill LJ, Pulsinelli WA, et al. Severe bilateral tremor in a liver transplant recipient taking cyclosporine. Mov Disord 1998;13(3):589–596.

5. Tarsy D, Indorf G. Tardive tremor due to metoclopramide. Mov Disord 2002;17(3):620–621.

6. Deuschl G, Schade-Brittinger C, Krack P, et al. A randomized trial of deep-brain stimulation for Parkinson's disease. N Engl J Med 2006;355(9):896–908.

7. Pahwa R, Factor SA, Lyons KE, et al. Practice parameter: treatment of Parkinson disease with motor fluctuations and dyskinesia (an evidence-based review): report of the Quality Standards Subcommittee of the American Academy of Neurology. Neurology 2006; 66(7):983–995.

8. Suchowersky O, Reich S, Perlmutter J, et al. Practice parameter: diagnosis and prognosis of new onset Parkinson disease (an evidence-based review): report of the Quality Standards Subcommittee of the American Academy of Neurology. Neurology 2006;66(7):968–975.

9. Zesiewicz TA, Elble R, Louis ED, et al. Practice parameter: therapies for essential tremor: report of the Quality Standards Subcommittee of the American Academy of Neurology. Neurology 2005;64(12): 2008–2020.

10. Hubble JP, Busenbark KL, Wilkinson S, et al. Deep brain stimulation for essential tremor. Neurology 1996;46(4):1150–1153.

11. Ondo WG. Essential tremor: treatment options. Curr Treat Options Neurol 2006;8(3):256–267.

12. Sechi G, Agnetti V, Sulas FM, et al. Effects of topiramate in patients with cerebellar tremor. Prog Neuropsychopharmacol Biol Psychiatry 2003;27(6):1023–1027.

13. Foote KD, Okun MS. Ventralis intermedius plus ventralis oralis anterior and posterior deep brain stimulation for posttraumatic Holmes tremor: two leads may be better than one: technical note. Neurosurgery 2005;56(2 Suppl):E445; discussion E.

14. Singer C, Papapetropoulos S, Spielholz NI. Primary writing tremor: report of a case successfully treated with botulinum toxin A injections and discussion of underlying mechanism. Mov Disord 2005;20(10): 1387–1388.

15. Ruzicka E, Jech R, Zarubova K, et al. VIM thalamic stimulation for tremor in a patient with IgM paraproteinaemic demyelinating neuropathy. Mov Disord 2003;18(10):1192–1195.

16. Penney SE, Bruce IA, Saeed SR. Botulinum toxin is effective and safe for palatal tremor: A report of five cases and a review of the literature. J Neurol 2006;253(7):857–860.

5

THE "SHUFFLING" PATIENT

PHENOMENOLOGY

A shuffling gait is a common complaint in any neurologic practice. The evaluation and diagnosis of a patient with gait abnormality can be challenging, and often depends on obtaining a comprehensive history and performing a careful neurologic evaluation. The etiology may be a result of a lesion anywhere in the neuraxis (extrapyramidal or not) or from a nonneurologic etiology, such as a rheumatologic disorder. The key to the diagnosis relies on the proper characterization of the gait and the recognition of associated neurologic symptoms.

Shuffling gait is usually seen in akinetic-rigid syndromes like Parkinson's disease (PD).

- It may be the initial complaint in non–tremor-predominant PD patients.

- Other conditions that may present shuffling of gait include, e.g., multiple systems atrophy (MSA), progressive supranuclear palsy (PSP), corticobasal ganglionic degeneration (CBGD), dementia with Lewy bodies (DLB), normal pressure hydrocephalus (NPH), some dementing processes, and frontal lobe syndromes.

- The characteristic shuffling patient adopts a stooped posture, with flexion of the neck and shoulders.

    - Steps are short, with slow speed.

- The trunk is flexed and rigid, and the knees tend to be flexed. However, the PSP patient often adopts a more erect trunk posture.

- The PD patient usually has asymmetric arm swing, compared with the other parkinsonian disorders.

  - Festination, defined as a tendency to increase velocity but with shorter steps, may also be seen in the shuffling patient, and is a characteristic finding in PD.

- Symptoms accompanying parkinsonism usually are the ones that give a clue to diagnosis. For example:

  - When shuffling gait is associated with urinary incontinence and cognitive impairment, NPH should be considered.

  - When shuffling gait is associated with early falls and vertical ophthalmoplegia, PSP should be considered.

  - When cognitive impairment occurs early, DLB, CBGD, and PSP should be considered.

  - Prominent autonomic dysfunction suggests MSA.

  - Likewise, marked dysequilibrium early in the disease is more suggestive of either PSP or MSA.

- Other gait abnormalities that may also present with shuffling are:

  - In isolated gait ignition failure, the patient often presents with difficulty initiating gait and frequent freezing with ambulation, aggravated when turning. The patient usually possesses normal postural responses but may have mild parkinsonian symptoms.

  - In frontal gait disorder, the patient gives the appearance of having the feet "glued" or "magnetized" to the floor. It is very difficult to initiate gait, and when gait is initiated, it may be shuffling in nature. Special maneuvers, like turning, may exacerbate the symptoms. This syndrome could result from extensive, bilateral ischemic white matter disease (atherosclerotic/vascular parkinsonism), hydrocephalus, or other frontal lobe disorders. This disorder has also been called gait apraxia.

EXAMINATION OF THE PATIENT

Once a comprehensive history is obtained, careful evaluation of gait should be performed (Table 5.1).

- Observe trunk posture while walking. The patient's pace, stance, stride, initiation, and performance in special maneuvers (such as turning repeatedly) should be noted.

- Ask the patient to stand up from a sitting position without pushing from the armrest. While failure to stand without assistance could result from proximal muscle weakness of the lower extremities (such as a myopathic condition), the same problem is often appreciated in moderate and severe stages of parkinsonism.

- Ask the patient to initiate walking. It should be an easy, free-flowing process.

- Hesitation in starting gait is suggestive of an akinetic-rigid syndrome.

- Once gait is initiated, stride, stance, and velocity should be noted. Shuffling steps are suggestive of akinetic-rigid syndromes, and may range in severity from very short steps to complete inability to ambulate (magnetic feet).

TABLE 5.1
Important Aspects of Gait Evaluation

Gait Aspect	Characteristics
Posture	Stooped versus upright
Stance	Narrow vs wide-based
Speed	Slow vs normal; with or without festination
Stride	Short, normal, or long
Gait initiation	Is there hesitation? Is it "magnetic"?
Freezing	Is there freezing during gait ignition or while turning?
Symptom asymmetry	Is the parkinsonism symmetrical versus asymmetrical?
Heel-toe walking	Look for truncal ataxia, cerebellar features
Postural reflexes	Early versus late onset
Falls	Backwards or forward; early vs late-onset

- A wide-based gait or difficulty in heel-toe walking suggests a concomitant cerebellar disorder, such as an olivopontocerebellar (OPCA) type of MSA or truncal ataxia.

- The patient should be observed in special maneuvers like turning in a corner or when suddenly asked to change direction. This may provoke the patient to "freeze" or may worsen the shuffling.

- The examiner should pay attention to symptom asymmetry or development of tremors, which are features suggestive of PD.

- Postural reflexes should then be examined, and this is usually performed by standing behind the patient and giving the patient a good tug on the shoulders.

- Examine for rigidity, bradykinesia, tremors.

- Look for associated features such as: apraxia, ataxia, sensory abnormalities, aphasia, cognitive impairment, and hyperreflexia.

PARKINSON'S DISEASE (see also Chapter 4)

- Parkinson's disease was first formally described by James Parkinson in an 1817 report.

- Parkinson described tremor, gait disorder, and bradykinesia, which he confused with paralysis, contributing to the misnomer *paralysis agitans*.

Epidemiology

- Estimating exactly how many people have Parkinson's disease is difficult because of inaccuracy in diagnosis and difficulty distinguishing the actual time of onset of PD.

- Between 750,000 and 1.5 million people in United States are estimated to have PD.

- There are between 4 and 20 new cases per 100,000 population per year. The incidence and prevalence of PD increase with age. About 2% of people over 65 years have PD.

- The average age of onset of symptoms is approximately 60 years.

- PD is more common in white people, less common in West Africa, and intermediate in China. African Americans and the Chinese in Taiwan have higher rates of Parkinson's disease than their counterparts in West Africa or China, suggesting that environmental factors may play a role.

- Men have a 1.5 times greater risk of developing PD compared to women.

- PD is called *young-onset* if it occurs between the ages of 21 and 40 years and *juvenile-onset* when symptoms start before 21 years of age.

- There is uncertainty about the effect of PD on survival. The estimated standardized mortality rate (the ratio of number of deaths in PD patients to controls) varies between 1.5 and 2.4.

    - Only half of death certificates in PD patients include PD as an underlying condition or contributory cause, as PD itself is not the direct cause of death. The primary cause of death is most commonly a secondary complication such as bronchopneumonia.

    - Earlier death is associated with dementia and later death with disease onset.

    - Although younger patients with PD have a longer absolute survival from diagnosis to death, the disease has a greater influence on survival in younger patients because of their greater life expectancy.

    - Tremor-predominant patients have better survival than those without tremor. Tremor-dominant patients also have better survival compared to patients with postural instability and gait disturbance.

Etiology

- The cause of PD remains unknown.

- Genetic, environmental, and an interaction between environmental risk factors and genetic susceptibility are all possible.

- PD may not be a single disease entity. The clinical presentation of PD may be caused by several different conditions.

Risk Factors

- Increasing age is the largest risk factor for developing PD; followed by a family history of PD.

- Other reported risk factors include higher education; occupation[1] (physicians and health-care workers); head trauma; exposure to herbicides, insecticides, and heavy metals; living in rural areas; drinking well water.[2]

Genetic Factors

- The majority of PD cases are sporadic, but a few are inherited (especially for PD presenting before age 50).

- If an individual has a family history of PD, the risk of developing PD is doubled compared to the rate in the background population. Between 15 and 20% of patients have a positive family history of PD.

- Gene mutations implicated in the development of PD include gene loci *PARK 1–11*. Some are autosomal dominant (AD) and others are recessive (AR).

    - *PARK 1* (AD), located on chromosome 4q21-q23, encodes for the protein alpha-synuclein, and is associated with Lewy bodies (the pathologic hallmark of PD and Lewy body dementia). This was first described in an Italian American family originating from Contursi and subsequently found in several families from Greece and elsewhere. Clinically, patients have onset of symptoms at an earlier age and are less likely to have tremor.

    - *PARK 2* (AR), located on chromosome 6q25.2-q27, encodes for the parkin protein, and Lewy bodies are absent. This was first described in a Japanese family, and patients can have an early or juvenile onset, a symmetrical presentation, more levodopa-induced dyskinesia, and slower disease progression. Excess psychiatric symptoms, early dystonia, and hyperreflexia which were previously considered to be clinical indicators of *parkin*-associated PD, but may correlate better with younger age of onset rather than the *parkin* mutation. However, in a recent report from China, the phenotype of slow progression, diurnal variation with sleep benefit, and hyperreflexia was relatively prominent. Mutations in *parkin* account for around 50% of AR young-onset familial PD and should be considered in cases with a family history consistent with AR inheritance and disease onset before the age of 45.

    - *PARK 3* (AD), located on chromosome 2p13, is associated with later onset (average age 59 years), cognitive impairment, levodopa responsiveness, and Lewy bodies are present. It has been identified in kindreds from northern Europe.

- *PARK 4* (AD) has now been mapped to *PARK 1* (chromosome 4q21)—affected individuals have doubling of alpha-synuclein expression (there is a triplication of the alpha-synuclein gene giving four copies of the usual gene rather than 2) and more extensive Lewy body pathology. Clinically, autonomic dysfunction, dementia, and weight loss occur in conjunction with parkinsonism.

- *PARK 5*—there is a mutation in the gene encoding ubiquitin carboxyterminal hydrolase L1 (*UCH-L1*) (probably AD)—this has only been reported in two German siblings who have an missense mutation in this gene, and it may be an extremely rare form of familial PD with incomplete penetrance; however, since the original report of these two cases in 1998, there have been no other kindreds with this mutation (193M in the *UCH-L1* gene). A more recent report suggests that *UCHL-1* is not a PD-susceptibility gene.

- *PARK 6* (AR), located on chromosome 1p35-p36, encodes for the PINK 1 protein and is associated with early age of onset and slower disease progression. It was first identified in an Italian family from Sicily from which four family members developed PD between the ages of 32 and 48 years. Functional imaging using positron emission tomography shows a more uniform pattern of reduced uptake in the caudate and putamen and a greater degree of dopamine loss than would have been expected from the clinical severity.

- *PARK 7* (AR), located on chromosome 1p36, is associated with early onset, slow disease progression, psychiatric disturbance, and dystonic features (e.g., blepharospasm). There is a mutation in the *DJ-1* gene and cells lacking in *DJ-1* appear to be more susceptible to oxidative stress.

- *PARK 8* (AD), located on chromosome 12p11.2-q13.1. Average onset at age is 51 years and clinically very similar to typical PD with unilateral onset and levodopa responsiveness. Foot dystonia may be present prior to and during drug therapy. Overall, patients do not report drug-induced dyskinesia. Pathology is variable. One case from a Lincolnshire, UK, kindred had loss of the pigmented neurons and gliosis of the substantia nigra and typical Lewy bodies. However, nigral degeneration without Lewy bodies was reported in the original description from Japan. A novel gene *LRRK2* (leucine-rich, repeat kinase 2), which encodes for the protein dardarin, has been identified as the gene responsible. The frequency of the *LRRK2* mutation is around 5% in cases of familial PD (based on a series of 118 familial PD patients—patients with one or more affected first-degree relative) and 1–2% in sporadic PD.

- *PARK 9* (AR—phenotype is unlike PD). Features are of pallido-pyramidal degeneration, supranuclear gaze paresis, and dementia.

- *PARK 10* (unknown). Fifty-one Icelandic families were genotyped and a susceptibility locus for late-onset PD was identified.

- *PARK 11* (AD). This locus was identified from genome-wide linkage analysis in a large multicenter study in the United States. No definite phenotype or inheritance has been reported.

Mitochondrial Inheritance

- A deficiency of mitchondrial complex I has been found which may result in a mitochondrial gene defect.

- Transmission through the maternal line was considered likely (as mitochondrial genes are maternally inherited). But in two separate studies, probands were more likely to report an affected father than an affected mother (which is clearly contrary to maternal inheritance).

Environmental Factors

- Toxins

  - MPTP. A chemistry graduate in San Francisco manufactured a pethidine analogue for street sale which was contaminated with MPTP (1-methyl-4-phenyl-1,2,3,6-tetrahydropyridine). Intravenous drug users injecting this product developed severe parkinsonism and active neuronal loss was found at autopsy.

  - Compounds structurally similar to MPTP are found in pesticides; small case-control studies show a small increased risk of parkinsonism in rural areas and farms, and in those who drink well water, but population-based controlled studies fail to show any association.

- Heavy metals. Manganese poisoning produces parkinsonism, but the clinical and pathologic features may be different from idiopathic PD.

  - In manganese intoxication, early psychiatric problems (mental irritability, compulsive actions, and hallucinations) occur, dystonia is more frequent, and tremor tends to be postural.

  - People living in Guam who consumed water containing aluminium and had low dietary intake of magnesium and calcium developed a parkinsonism-dementia complex. A separate theory suggested that the syndrome was caused by a plant neurotoxin from cycad flour.

  - Iron may enhance free radical formation causing lipid peroxidation and cell death.

- Carbon monoxide

  - Parkinsonism is a delayed effect and has features of bradykinesia, rigidity, and occasional resting tremor. Dystonia and emotional changes may also be present. Another variant is of akinetic mutism.

- Infections

  - In the early 1900s, postencephalitic parkinsonism raised the possibility of an infective (probably viral) etiology. The acute phase of the disease usually lasts several weeks and the clinical picture is of pronounced somnolence and ophthalmoplegia. The parkinsonian syndrome presents months or years following infection (average 25 years, median 5 years). However, the clinical and pathologic features of postencephalitic parkinsonism are different from those of idiopathic PD. In postencephalitic parkinsonism, clinically progression is slow and pathologically there are Alzheimer-type neurofibrillary tangles, whereas in PD there is a progressive disorder and histologically there are Lewy bodies.

- Emotional stress

  - An increased risk of PD in people who have endured extreme psychologic and physical stress has been reported.

It is postulated that emotional stress increases dopamine turnover causing oxidative nerve cell death. This is unproven.

- Personality

  - Premorbid personality traits of shyness, being more introverted, and depression have been associated with an increased risk of PD. In retrospective studies, PD patients were more cautious, less flexible, and quieter compared to control subjects. This needs to be examined in larger studies.

Clinical Progression

- Clinical signs and symptoms develop once there is at least 50% depletion of striatal dopamine (estimated from imaging studies). However, there may be as much as 60–80% loss of pigmented neurons in the substantia nigra (compensatory mechanisms may affect the scan appearance and thereby account for the discrepancy).

- The preclinical phase of the disease may be one to several years, but this is unknown.

- The rates of disease progression vary between individuals. Some tremor-dominant patients progress very slowly.

- Ten to 20% of patients have no tremor and remain akinetic-rigid or have primarily a gait disorder.

- When patients commence treatment, there is usually an improvement in the motor function score. The response to levodopa is often dose related. Untreated patients have a total Unified Parkinson's Disease Rating Scale (UPDRS) score deterioration of about 13 points per year.

- Motor complications (wearing off, involuntary movements, and the "on/off" effect) are traditionally stated to occur in 50% of patients after 5 years on levodopa treatment, although lower rates than this are described in several studies. In general, dopamine agonist monotherapy is associated with lower motor complication rates.

- For patients on levodopa, 40% remain free of dyskinesia after 5 years versus 70% who are free of dyskinesia if on the dopamine agonist treatment. However, levodopa is a more efficacious treatment in terms of improvement in motor score.

- Young-onset patients (<40 years) develop motor complications earlier; occurring in almost 100% at 6 years.

- Patients who are older at symptom onset generally have a more rapid deterioration in motor features.

- Older age, early cognitive problems, associated comorbidities, presentation with rigidity and bradykinesia (i.e., lack of tremor at onset), decreased dopamine responsiveness, and greater baseline impairment are associated with poorer prognosis.

- Progression of disease may not be linear. Several studies suggest that the rate of decline is more rapid initially, then slows in the more advanced disease stages (however, the effects of treatment need to be considered, as this will influence interpretation of severity and progression rates).

Clinical Features

- The three cardinal motor features of PD are[3]:

  1. Bradykinesia

  2. Muscular rigidity

  3. Tremor (4- to 6-Hz rest tremor)

- To reach a diagnosis of PD, there must be bradykinesia and at a least one of the two other cardinal features.

- Postural instability (not caused by primary visual, vestibular, cerebellar, or proprioceptive dysfunction) is often included as a fourth or supporting feature.

- Asymmetry

  - Idiopathic PD is generally an asymmetric condition. The side of onset (left or right) does not have an association with a patient's hemisphere dominance (i.e., handedness).

  - Symptoms and signs remain worse on the side of onset throughout the disease course (including severity of motor fluctuations and dyskinesias).

- Bradykinesia

  - Bradykinesia is a slowness of initiating voluntary movement and sustaining repetitive movements with progressive reduction in speed and amplitude. Hypokinesia is poverty of movement.

- Patient symptoms and functional limitations which reflect bradykinesia/hypokinesia include:

  - Loss of arm swing

  - Difficulty with walking, a tendency to drag a leg in early disease

  - Increasingly small handwriting (micrographia)

  - Difficulty with fine hand movements—buttons, zippers, and cutting food

  - Difficulty turning in bed

  - Loss of facial expression, often described as a mask-like face (hypomimia)

  - Hypophonia (reduced voice volume and modulation)

- Bradykinesia causes significant disability affecting quality of life in PD patients which almost always responds to antiparkinsonian therapy.

- Rigidity

  - Rigidity is an involuntary increase in muscle tone and can affect all muscle groups. Rigidity is present throughout the range of movement and can be described as "lead-pipe" if smooth. "Cog-wheel" tremor is movement like a ratchet, and while there may be a subjective coexisting tremor which gives a feeling of cog-wheeling, true cog-wheeling is a form of rigidity independent of tremor.

  - Rigidity is tested for by passively moving the limb through normal movements.

  - Mild rigidity can be detected by "activation"; e.g., asking the patient to open and close the contralateral hand.

  - Patients describe rigidity as muscle stiffness or sometimes pain. Occasionally, patients initially present to an orthopedist with a frozen shoulder, which is actually the first sign of their PD. Pain in PD may also be caused by dystonia.

- Tremor

  - Rest tremor is typical of PD and occurs when the body part is relaxed; e.g., the arms and hands resting in the lap with the patient seated. Distraction may help "bring out" a rest tremor, especially if the patient is anxious; e.g., asking the patient to count backwards.

- Postural and action tremor can also be seen in PD.

- Tremor disappears during sleep.

- It is the presenting symptom of PD in 40–70% of cases, and between 68 and 100% of PD patients will have rest tremor at some point during the course of their illness. Ten to 20% of PD patients do not have tremor.

- Classically, tremor is at rest at a frequency of 4–6 Hz ("pill-rolling," as the tremor has a rotatory component), but the tremor can be at other frequencies.

- Tremor usually starts in one hand and arm, and progresses to the ipsilateral leg, later spreading contralaterally (tremor may, however, start in the leg).

- Postural tremor is often present. There is latency between rest and postural tremor, meaning that the patient's arm and hand show rest tremor, which disappears when taking up a posture (e.g., holding up the arms), then the tremor reemerges (hence sometimes called reemergent tremor).

- Chin, jaw, and eyelid tremor can also occur in PD, but tremor of the whole head is rare. Head tremor seen as nodding (yes-yes tremor) or shaking (no-no tremor) and is a feature of essential tremor rather than PD, and can rarely occur in PD. Head tremor can also occur in patients with cervical dystonia.

- Tremor is the often the most difficult symptom of the classic triad to treat. About half of cases will notice a treatment response with improvement in tremor, but tremor is seldom completely abolished. Patients are often troubled by the persistence of tremor despite therapy, and may report that the treatment is not working because tremor remains, even though bradykinesia has improved.

- Tremor of PD tends to increase with stress and anxiety, but this is not specific and is seen in many other types of tremor.

- Postural Instability

  - Patients report poor balance, unsteadiness, and falls.

  - Postural instability is examined using the pull test. The examiner stands behind the patient and pulls back sharply on the patient's shoulders (the feet should be slightly apart, unlike their position in a Romberg's test). Patients may correct themselves in the early stages (retropulsion— the patient may take two to three steps back, but can correct themselves), but in advanced stages, they fall if unsupported.

Misdiagnosis of PD

- Misdiagnosis is common and occurs in about 25–50% in community studies.

- Lower misdiagnosis rates (10–25%) occur in specialty centers, although this is based on diagnosis made later in the course of the disease (i.e., the last premortem visit diagnosis compared against autopsy results is likely to reveal more accurate clinical diagnosis compared against the initial diagnosis at presentation).

- It may take time for the diagnosis to emerge.

- PD is sometimes mistaken for primary depression (reduced facial expression, motor slowing, constipation), hypothyroidism, or slowing due to normal aging.

- *Striatal toe*: A cramp or muscle spasm in the forefoot, in which the great toe involuntary extends (dorsiflexes; i.e., points upwards) is sometimes the first sign of PD. Striatal toe is a form of dystonia, and when dystonia is the presenting feature of PD, the feet are involved in the vast majority of cases.

- *Frozen shoulder*: Unilateral frozen shoulder resulting from rigidity and bradykinesia is sometimes a presenting feature of PD.

- *Psychogenic movement disorder*: Early-onset PD, especially with any atypical features, is sometimes mislabeled as being psychogenic. *Psychogenic parkinsonism* is rare. Suggestive features include abrupt onset, rapid initial progression which plateaus, bizarre gait, exaggerated slowness, and psychologic overlay. The levodopa response varies between nil and excellent, but drug-induced motor complications and advancing complications (such as dementia) do not occur. Functional presynaptic dopamine imaging can help differentiate psychogenic (normal scan) from idiopathic PD (abnormal scan). Psychologic complications occur in PD, and some manifest physically such as tremor, hyperventilation, and other involuntary movements.

Motor Complications

Motor Fluctuations

- During the early stages of PD, treatment is usually uncompli-cated. With disease progression, there is the eventual appear-ance of motor fluctuations and dyskinesias, making the disease progress from a nondisabling to a disabling stage (Table 5.2).

- Twenty-eight to 84% of patients will develop motor fluctua-tions by 4–6 years after disease onset.

- Motor fluctuations decrease the quality of life of patients.

- With disease progression, patients develop greater sensitivity to small changes in levodopa levels (Figure 5.1).

- Treatment of motor fluctuations becomes a challenge in the later stages of Parkinson's disease.

Risk Factors

- Development of motor fluctuations is variable between sub-jects, suggesting that some patients may be predisposed to develop motor fluctuations early in the disease.

- Age of onset of disease—patients with young-onset PD are more likely to develop motor fluctuations than late-onset PD.

- Duration of treatment—the longer the patient has been on dopaminergic therapy, the more likely the patient is to de-velop motor fluctuations.

- Total daily dose—motor fluctuations are more likely to happen in patients taking higher dosages of levodopa or agonists.

TABLE 5.2
Motor Fluctuations Related to Levodopa Therapy

Wearing off

On-off fluctuations

Dose failures

Delayed on

Off dystonia

Falls

Freezing

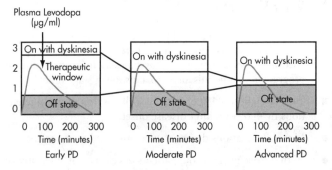

FIGURE 5.1

Changes in response to levodopa with time.

- Drug formulation—pulsatile versus continual dopaminergic stimulation (pulsatile dopaminergic stimulation may increase the risk and speed of development of motor fluctuations compared with more continuous dopaminergic stimulation [in primate studies]; human studies are underway).

- Food intake—meals with a large content of neutral amino acids may compete with levodopa for absorption, and contribute to delayed gastric emptying resulting in erratic absorption of levodopa.

Motor Fluctuations Associated with Levodopa Therapy

- Wearing off

    - Most common and usually the earliest motor fluctuation.

    - Decreased benefit from levodopa after each dose (less than usual 4 hours); it "wears off too early."

    - Drug benefit early in the disease is gradual and predictable, but as the disease advances, drug benefit may disappear unpredictably, and even sometimes suddenly.

    - Tremors, bradykinesia, rigidity begin to appear before the next dose.

    - Wearing off symptoms may also include nonmotor symptoms such as autonomic (flushing, sweating, lightheadedness), psychiatric (depression, anxiety, panic), cognitive (bradyphrenia), and sensory phenomena (abdominal, back or limb pain, paresthesias, fatigue).

- "Off" Period dystonia

  - Frequently early morning dystonia, but this symptom may also occur between dosages.

  - Foot cramps and toes curling are the most common manifestations.

  - Dystonic posturing of the arms and/or legs may also occur.

  - May be a source of pain for some patients, and they experience relief once they turn "on."

  - Some patients may experience back pain and shoulder pain (may even occur years before diagnosis).

- "On-Off" fluctuations

  - Refers to unpredictable, sometimes sudden fluctuations from a treated (or overtreated) state to an undertreated state (stiff and rigid alternates with dyskinetic).

  - Consists of periods of unpredictable, severe akinesia.

  - May last from minutes to hours.

  - Sometimes will not respond to further administration of levodopa. Apomorphine can be used as a rescue therapy. Changing medication intervals, doses, and adding agonists can be useful.

- Dose failure

  - Characterized by lack of benefit after drug ingestion.

  - Usually a complication of long-term therapy.

  - Probably secondary to GI mechanics (delayed gastric emptying, poor drug absorption).

- Freezing

- The patient has difficulty initiating gait, walking, or other movements.

- Start hesitation may be the most common form of freezing.

- May also present as gait ignition failure, turn hesitation, sudden freezing, or on-off freezing.

- Freezing can occur during on and off stages.

- It may be a source of great disability for patients, limiting mobility and causing frequent falls.

- On freezing can be very difficult to treat. Freezing in the off state may respond to medication optimization.

Motor Fluctuations Induced by Levodopa/Dopaminergic Therapy

- Dyskinesia

  - Usually consists of choreic or ballistic movements. Dystonia and myoclonus may also be appreciated.

  - It is usually worse on the side most affected by PD.

  - The onset usually affects the lower extremity, especially the foot.

  - Mild dyskinesia may not be apparent to the PD patient but can be concerning to the family.

  - Respiratory muscles may be involved in severe dyskinesias.

  - May be seen in two forms:

  1. Peak dose dyskinesia: Development of dyskinesias at the peak effect of the medications.

  2. Biphasic dyskinesia (dyskinesia-improvement-dyskinesias): After drug ingestion, dyskinesias are appreciated followed by maximal drug benefit which is then followed by dyskinesia as the benefit begins to subside.

- Dystonia

  - May occur with wearing-off.

  - Can also occur when levodopa levels are rising or falling.

  - Painful foot cramps are an example.

DIFFERENTIAL DIAGNOSIS (Table 5.3)

Vascular Parkinsonism

- Vascular parkinsonism accounts for 4–12% of all cases of parkinsonism, but a rate of 3–6% emerges if only studies using imaging or pathologic diagnostic data are included.

TABLE 5.3
Useful Clues in Differentiating Shuffling Patients

Syndrome	Clues to diagnosis
Parkinson's disease	Asymmetrical onset of symptoms, good response to levodopa, resting tremor is prominent
Progressive supranuclear palsy	Vertical gaze palsy, gait and balance disturbance early in the disease (usually falling backwards), axial rigidity, neck extension when walking, "surprised" look on the face, poor response to levodopa
Corticobasal ganglionic degeneration	Dementia, cortical sensory loss, ideomotor apraxia, "alien limb" syndrome, asymmetrical symptoms, poor response to levodopa
Multiple systems atrophy	Shy-Drager syndrome—early autonomic disturbance, orthostatic hypotension, neuropathy, constipation, erectile dysfunction; may have some response to levodopa, early gait disturbance
	Olivopontocerebellar atrophy—cerebellar signs; may have some response to levodopa
	Striatonigral degeneration—laryngeal stridor; may have some response to levodopa
Normal pressure hydrocephalus	Triad of cognitive impairment, gait abnormality, and urinary incontinence
Lewy body disease	Hallucinations early in the disease, dementia, fluctuation of symptoms; paradoxical worsening with medications
Vascular parkinsonism	May be gradual or sudden-onset parkinsonism; with vascular risk factors such as diabetes, hypertension; usually small-vessel ischemic disease

■ The incidence and prevalence of vascular parkinsonism increase with age, and it is more common in men than women.

■ The pattern typically involves the lower body (as compared to idiopathic PD in which the arms and upper body are more often initially affected). However, the upper body can be involved. Patients with vascular parkinsonism are more likely to be older, have postural instability, a history of falling, dementia, corticospinal findings, and incontinence.[4]

■ The original description by Critchley in the 1920s was of a predominant gait disorder (short steps—*march a petit pas*) with additional features of dementia and pyramidal signs. Classically, the presentation was described as an acute onset, which was symmetrical, without tremor, but with postural instability and a poor response to dopamine replacement therapy. However, the onset is more commonly insidious.

In one series, only about a quarter of cases of vascular parkinsonism were considered to have an acute onset with a new ischemic stroke event, but even here the new event may have unmasked an insidious process.

■ There is, therefore, some suggestion that there may be two types of vascular parkinsonism:

1. With acute onset possibly associated with basal ganglia infarction.

2. With a more insidious onset, possibly associated with more diffuse subcortical white matter ischemia.

■ Vascular risk factors including hypertension and diabetes increase the risk of developing vascular parkinsonism. Other common vascular risk factors including a family history of vascular disease, other evidence of vascular disease (ischemic heart disease or peripheral vascular disease), hypercholesterolemia, and smoking would seem likely to increase the risk of vascular parkinsonism, but evidence is lacking. A history of stroke is also a risk factor.

■ Structural imaging may show basal ganglia infarcts, subcortical ischemia, or more diffuse small vessel changes. These findings support the diagnosis of vascular parkinsonism, but can of course also be present in the absence of clinical parkinsonism.

■ In one series, about 10% of cases with a basal ganglia stroke went on to develop vascular parkinsonism, but in another study, 38% of patients with lacunar basal ganglia infarcts on magnetic resonance imaging (MRI) had clinical features of parkinsonism.

■ Functional imaging using single photon emission computed tomography (SPECT) or positron emission tomography (PET) to check the integrity of presynaptic neurons is abnormal in idiopathic PD, but normal in vascular parkinsonism (unless there is focal basal ganglia infarction).

■ There are three pathologic patterns of vascular parkinsonism:

1. Multiple lacunar infarcts clinically associated with gait disorder, pyramidal deficits, cognitive impairment, and pseudobulbar palsy.

2. Subcortical arteriosclerotic encephalopathy (Binswanger's disease) clinically associated with a progressive gait disorder and dementia.

3. Basal ganglia infarct (usually lacunar); this type is rare.

- Idiopathic Parkinson's disease and vascular parkinsonism are relatively common in an aging population and can coexist.

- Addressing vascular risk—control of hypertension, diabetes, hypercholesterolemia, considering antiplatelet therapy, and advising smoking cessation seem sensible, although these therapeutic strategies have not been studied in vascular parkinsonism.

- Typically, there is a poor therapeutic response to levodopa in vascular parkinsonism, but some evidence of a levodopa response in patients with pathologic confirmation of vascular parkinsonism was noted in a case review (12 of 17 patients had a good or excellent response documented). In clinical practice, it is appropriate to try levodopa, often up to the maximum tolerated dose, and continue treatment if there is clinical benefit, but discontinue it if there is no response, or if adverse effects outweigh any benefit.

Multiple System Atrophy

- Multiple system atrophy (MSA) is a syndrome that may manifest with parkinsonism, autonomic dysfunction, and cerebellar features, or alternatively a combination. The age-adjusted prevalence of MSA is about 4 per 100,000 persons.

  - Parkinsonism

    - Bradykinesia, rigidity, postural instability, and tremor. In the consensus statement for the diagnosis of MSA, bradykinesia plus one feature of rigidity, postural instability, or tremor are required to meet diagnostic criteria.

    - Tremor is present in two-thirds of patients with multiple system atrophy, but often not prominent or only seen initially. Less than 10% have the pill-rolling rest tremor which is typical of idiopathic PD. The tremor of MSA can be of an irregular jerky type, noted during both posture and action; and may be due to myoclonic jerks, which are sometimes touch or stretch sensitive.

  - Autonomic problems

    - Falls (relating to orthostatic hypotension, a fall of over 20 systolic and over 10 diastolic within 3 minutes of standing or head-up tilt, and low resting blood pressure).

- Impotence and early erectile dysfunction.

- Bladder instability (urinary incontinence or incomplete bladder emptying).

- Cerebellar signs

  - Gait ataxia

  - Speech problems (ataxic dysarthria)

  - Nystagmus (although this is not common)

  - Incoordination

  - Pyramidal signs can also occur

    - Brisk reflexes

    - Upgoing (extensor) plantar reflexes

- Patients whose presentation is predominantly parkinsonian are labeled as having the MSA-P subtype (formerly known as striatonigral degeneration) of MSA, while those with stronger cerebellar features are classified as having subtype MSA-C (formerly called sporadic olivopontocerebellar atrophy).

- MSA-P is between two and four times commoner than MSA-C.

- The mean age of onset is 54 years (younger than idiopathic PD), and there are no known pathologically proven cases with symptoms developing before the age of 30 years.

- Dyskinesia can develop, especially the orofacial type.

- Dementia is uncommon. In the consensus diagnostic categories and exclusion criteria for MSA, the *Diagnostic and Statistical Manual of Mental Disorders (*DSM) criteria for dementia is considered an exclusion criterion for MSA. However, alterations of personality and mood can occur.

Progressive Supranuclear Palsy

- The median age of onset is 60–65 years.

- The median disease duration from diagnosis to death varies between 5.9 and 9.7 years.

- The age-adjusted prevalence is about 6/100,000.

- Parkinsonism occurs, particularly axial rigidity (hence neck and trunk movements are more affected than limbs).

- Early falls (with a tendency to fall backwards, "like a tree trunk").

- Loss of vertical eye movement (unable to look up or down on command but able to follow a moving target in early stages).

- Speech and swallowing difficulty.

- Dementia.

- Upper motor neuron signs.

- Neurofibrillary tangles and neuropil threads in the basal ganglia and other parts of the brain stem and tau-positive tufts are the pathologic features.[5]

Corticobasal Degeneration

- Parkinsonism occurs along with cortical dysfunction.

- Parkinsonism manifests as an akinetic-rigid syndrome which is unresponsive to levodopa.

- Cognitive impairment is a dominant feature.

- Symptoms usually start after the age of 60.

- Unilateral bradykinesia and rigidity occur with or without tremor.

- An irregular jerky arm is typical.

- Progressive gait disturbance, dystonia, dysphagia, and dysarthria may occur.

- Features include apraxia (patients complain that their limb does not understand tasks and the patient has difficulty peforming skilled movements), cortical sensory loss, and memory loss.

- Other signs include myoclonus, corticospinal signs, choreoathetosis, supranuclear gaze abnormalities, and blepharospasm.

- Symptoms spread contralaterally within 1 year.

- Patients may have an "alien" limb; e.g., if they are scratching, they deny that it is their own hand being used.

- The cause is unknown, but there is an accumulation of the tau protein.[6,7]

- Structural neuroimaging shows cortical atrophy and functional neuroimaging shows reduced cortical blood flow in the frontoparietotemporal area, which is sometimes asymmetric.

- There is no specific treatment, and supportive multidisciplinary care is required.

- Pharmacotherapy may include antidepressants and a trial of dopaminergic therapy. Clonazepam may help myoclonus, and baclofen can be used for muscle spasm.

Wilson's Disease (see also Chapter 6)

- A genetic (autosomal recessive) disorder with a deficiency of a copper-carrier membrane protein. The abnormal gene is located on chromosome 13.

- Should be considered in all young (<50 years) patients presenting with parkinsonism.

- Fifty percent of patients present with neurologic or psychiatric symptoms, and the remainder present with symptoms of liver disease usually in childhood (up to age 53).

- Serum ceruloplasmin is low and urinary copper is raised.

- Kayser-Fleischer ring (a brown deposit in the cornea, around the outer edge of the iris, which represents a depostion of copper in Descemet's membrane).

  - May be seen by naked eye, especially in patients with blue irises.

  - Usually requires an ophthalmologic slit-lamp examination.

- Treatment is with penicillamine or other copper-chelating agents.[8]

Dementia with Lewy Bodies

- Dementia with Lewy bodies account for about 20% of all dementia.

- May present as a predominant dementia with some extrapyramidal signs or initially as parkinsonism with early-onset dementia. The term *Parkinson's disease with dementia* (PDD) has been used when parkinsonism predates the development of dementia by at least 1 year, and dementia with Lewy bodies (DLB) when dementia starts before that.

- Visual hallucinations, delusions, and psychosis may occur in the absence of dopaminergic therapy.

- Cognitive decline is progressive but may fluctuate (there are lucid periods when mental performance is much nearer normal).

- The Scientific Issues Committee of the Movement Disorder society task force formed consensus criteria for the clinical diagnosis of dementia with Lewy bodies. To reach a *possible* diagnosis the inclusion criteria are:

  - Progressive cognitive decline of sufficient magnitude to interfere with normal social or occupational function (prominent or persistent memory impairment may not necessarily occur in the early stages but is usually evident with progression; deficits on tests of attention and frontal-subcortical skills and visuospatial ability may be especially prominent).

  - One of three core features:

    - Fluctuating cognition with pronounced variations in attention and alertness

    - Recurrent visual hallucinations

    - Parkinsonism

  - Supportive criteria are:

    - Repeated falls

    - Syncope

    - Transient loss of consciousness

    - Neuroleptic sensitivity

    - Systematized delusions, hallucinations in other modalities (e.g., hearing voices or feeling the touch of a visualized figure)

    - Depression

    - Rapid eye movement sleep behavior disorder

  - To reach a *probable* diagnosis of dementia with Lewy bodies patients need to fulfill the *possible* criteria plus one more core features.

  - Management often involves reduction and sometimes discontinuation of antiparkinson medication—particularly anticholinergics, selegiline, amantadine, and dopamine agonists. The newer atypical neuroleptics (e.g., quetiapine) may be considered. Cognitive function may improve with cholinesterase inhibitors. Dopamine agonists in conjunction with atypical neuroleptics have sometimes been used successfully.

Normal Pressure Hydrocephalus

- Despite its popularity, normal pressure hydrocephalus (NPH) is a rather rare condition in which parkinsonism is associated with "normal pressure" hydrocephalus and primary empty sella.

- In addition to parkinsonism, symptoms are of urinary incontinence, gait disturbance, and dementia.

- It is distinguished from PD by:

  - Rigidity, tremor, and bradykinesia tending to be less common than in PD.

  - There being a limited, if any, response to levodopa.

  - Incontinence is usually urinary, but may also be bowel incontinence.

  - Dementia may progress less rapidly than in Alzheimer's disease or in Parkinson's disease dementia.

- Structural neuroimaging aids diagnosis.

- Surgical shunting should be considered. However, the risks of surgery may outweigh potential benefit, particularly when poor prognostic features including dementia, long-standing symptoms, and cortical atrophy are present.[9]

- NPH may be confused with Parkinson's disease or vascular dementia. Many experts feel NPH is overdiagnosed and caution should be exercised before consideration of high risk surgical procedures such as shunting.

Drug-induced Parkinsonism

- In some epidemiologic studies, between a third and a half of parkinsonism is caused by medication.

- Drug-induced parkinsonism is sometimes difficult to distinguish from idiopathic PD, but certain features are helpful and the drug history is crucial.

- Although symptoms may be asymmetrical, drug-induced parkinsonism often presents symmetrically.

- Neuroleptics are most commonly implicated (the newer atypical neuroleptics are less likely to induce parkinsonism, but still often cause milder forms of parkinsonism). In one prevalence study, 62% of patients on neuroleptics developed movement disorders, encompassing a mix of akathisia (31%), parkinsonism (23%), and tardive dyskinesia (32%).

- Antinausea agents (e.g., prochlorperazine, metoclopramide, cinnarizine) are other common culprits.

- Sodium valproate and tetrabenazine cause parkinsonism but at much lower rates. Antidepressants and calcium antagonists have been implicated largely through case reports but data are not robust. As depression is common in PD, antidepressants can often be helpful, and worsening parkinsonism is seldom an issue in clinical practice.

- Although the parkinsonism usually improves on withdrawal of the offending drug, this may take many months and sometimes symptoms persist. If they persist, and especially if they worsen, for about 6 months or more after drug withdrawal, PD may have been unmasked (i.e., induced earlier than if the offending drug had not been prescribed).

- Drug-unmasked PD may be distinguished from pure drug-induced parkinsonism using presynaptic functional dopamine imaging (PET or SPECT), which is abnormal in PD but normal in drug-induced parkinsonism. Most cases of drug-induced parkinsonism that persist represent unmasked PD.

Essential Tremor (see also Chapter 4)

- In early disease, the main differential from Parkinson's disease is essential tremor (ET).

- ET is approximately 10 times more common than PD.

- Men and women are equally affected by essential tremor.

- The tremors of ET and PD are usually distinguished on clinical examination. Rest tremor is usually not present in ET. The tremor frequency of ET is similar to that of the latent postural tremor of PD, but can be faster (4–12 Hz). In ET, there is no latency on taking up a posture (i.e., the tremor starts as soon as a movement is initiated). The tremor of ET is generally in the plane of flexion/extension, whereas in PD, there is also rotatory movement (e.g., at the wrist; hence the classic description of "pill-rolling" tremor).

- In essential tremor:

  - Tremor is usually bilateral and occurs with posture and action tremor compared with the asymmetrical rest tremor of PD.

  - Family history is positive in approximately 50% of cases (there is an autosomal dominant mode if inheritance).

  - Tremor improves with alcohol (the benefit of alcohol is more than merely the anxiolytic effect of alcohol).

  - Tremor begins at a younger age (however, the incidence of ET increases with age).

  - Tremor is usually present for some time (often years), progresses considerably more slowly than PD, and is not associated with other parkinsonian features.

  - Tremor of the head and neck is common in ET, whereas in PD, head tremor is rare but chin and lip tremor do occur.

  - In idiopathic PD, tremor is usually asymmetrical, starts unilaterally, and occurs at rest, a positive family history is much less likely, the tremor does not generally respond to alcohol, other PD features (rigidity and bradykinesia) are present, and the symptoms are usually more rapidly progressive.

- Essential tremor may not need pharmacologic treatment, and an accurate diagnosis and reassurance are sometimes sufficient. In moderate to severe cases, beta blockers may improve the tremor. If beta blockers are ineffective, contra-indicated, or cause adverse effects, primidone can be tried alone or in combination (but can cause sedation and behavioural effects). Other treatments such as gabapentin and topiramate have some clinical trial evidence of benefit (although only small numbers of topiramate-treated cases completed the study).[10] In severe intractable cases, surgery such as thalamotomy or deep brain stimulation should be considered.[11]

DIAGNOSTIC WORKUP (Table 5.4)

Treatment

Motor Aspects: Management Principles

- Currently available drug treatments provide symptomatic benefit; none has proven to be neuroprotective.

TABLE 5.4
Diagnosis/Workup of Common Parkinsonian Syndromes

Is there history of exposure to dopamine receptor blocking agents?	If yes, consider drug-induced parkinsonism	Symptoms usually symmetrical
Is there history of cerebrovascular disease?	Consider vascular parkinsonism, especially if symptoms symmetric	Lower body parkinsonism is usually a presentation of vascular parkinsonism
Is the patient <50 years old	Evaluate for Wilson's disease	Serum ceruloplasmin, 24-hr urine copper excretion; slit-lamp evaluation; if needed, liver biopsy
Abnormal MRI of brain	Consider: Vascular parkinsonism Assess for NPH Toxic/metabolic (hypoxic anoxic injury, manganese intoxication, iron deposition)	Basal ganglia or periventricular ischemic gliotic changes Ventriculomegaly Increased signal in BG
"Normal" MRI of brain	PD	Slowly progressive, levodopa responsive, asymmetrical, resting tremors
	MSA	Autonomic disturbances, poor levodopa response; MRI may show atrophic pons
	PSP	Early falls, dysphagia, poor levodopa response, vertical gaze paresis; MRI may show small midbrain
	CBGD	Asymmetric, dystonia, alien hand, poor levodopa response, dystonia; MRI/SPECT scan may show cortical asymmetry especially the temporal lobes
	LBD	Early hallucinations, poor levodopa response, memory disturbances, fluctuations in mental status

BG, basal ganglia; CBGD, corticobasal ganglionic degeneration; LBD, Lewy body dementia; MSA, multiple system atrophy; NPH, normal pressure hydrocephalus; PSP, progressive supranuclear palsy.

- Treatment is initiated when required from a functional viewpoint (this is variable between patients, and the decision requires patient and often caregiver input).

- Treatment is started at a variable point after the onset of symptoms, but usually 2–5 years (note symptom onset usually predates diagnosis).

- There are several initial treatment choices, each with advantages and disadvantages. The main choices are levodopa (with decarboxylase inhibitor), dopamine agonists, and monoamine oxidase B inhibitors. Anticholinergics and amantadine are also sometimes used. Drug choice is patient-specific depending on comorbidities, biologic age, and patient choice. Several randomized clinical trials compare drug classes; e.g., levodopa versus dopamine agonists, monoamine oxidae B (MAOB) inhibitors versus placebo.

- PD is not a "static" illness. Therefore, medications need to be titrated over time.

- In general, it is best to find the lowest dosage of any PD medication that will provide functional improvement.

- Not all motor symptoms of PD respond uniformly to pharmacologic treatment. Bradykinesia and rigidity are most responsive to medications; postural instability is the least responsive to treatment; and pharmacologic response to tremor is variable.

- When to increase or add in therapy:

  - Signs of disease progression are increasing slowness, stiffness, and worsening tremor.

  - Initial low-dose therapy with dopamine agonist or levodopa is generally increased gradually for worsening symptoms and levels of function.

  - Once initial therapy reaches the recommended maximum dose or maximally tolerated level, and addition of a second agent is required, a drug from a different class will become appropriate.

- Signs of overtreatment:

  - Dopaminergic excess is characterized by confusion, hallucinations, and involuntary movement (dyskinesia).

  - Reduction of the dopaminergic therapy lowers such side effects, but many patients prefer to tolerate mild visual hallucinations or dyskinesia as they find off periods unpleasant and sometimes painful.

- Excessive sleep is common to all dopaminergic therapy and is dose related, and appropriate caution driving or operating machinery is needed.

- Sudden onset of sleep can occur rarely, more with dopamine agonists, and necessitates stopping driving and using machinery.

Drugs Used to Treat Motor Fluctuations

- Levodopa

  - Levodopa is a naturally occurring amino acid found in seedlings, pods, and broadbeans.

  - Levodopa was first introduced in the early 1970s and was a major therapeutic advance.

  - Initially very high levodopa doses were used, and peripheral metabolism to dopamine caused intolerable nausea, dizziness, and postural hypotension, limiting the use of the drug.

  - The discovery of peripheral decarboxylase inhibitors (carbidopa or benserazide) led to combined products of levodopa with decarboxylase inhibitors which dramatically alleviated adverse peripheral dopaminergic effects.

  - Levodopa remains the most effective treatment for parkinsonian symptom control and remains the "gold standard."

  - Levodopa is available in many forms and formulations. Similar preparation names containing different amounts of active ingredients necessitate care by prescribers. At least 70 mg per day of the carbidopa is necessary to completely block peripheral decarboxylation (smaller doses have increased side effects).

  - The dosing is typically initiated at one 25/100 mg carbidopa/levodopa tablet three times daily and increased as necessary until clinical response is achieved. The recommended maximum dose of levodopa per day is 2000 mg.

  - The main problems with levodopa result from a short half-life (90 minutes), which leads to peaks and troughs in serum (and therefore brain) levodopa levels causing pulsatile rather than the more physiologic continuous dopaminergic stimulation.

- The controlled-release preparations of levodopa were developed to prolong the duration of action and provide smoother control and lessen the development of motor complications.

  - Sinemet CR is designed to release active ingredients over a 4- to 6-hour period via a slowly dissolving polymeric matrix and has approximately 70% bioavailability compared to standard (immediate) release.

  - Up to 30% more levodopa per day may be necessary, and dosing interval can be increased by up to 30%.

  - In clinical trials, there was no difference in the development of motor fluctuations between immediate and controlled-release preparations.

  - The controlled-release levodopa preparations may be subject to more variable gut absorption than immediate-release preparations, which can contribute to fluctuations in advanced disease.

  - Controlled-release levodopa has a place as a nocturnal dose to help reduce overnight symptoms (dopamine agonists also have this role due to their longer half-life).

  - Parcopa is an immediate-release, rapidly dissolving oral carbidopa/levodopa preparation available in the doses of immediate-release carbidopa/levodopa. It dissolves in the mouth without requiring water. However, its absorption is still intestinal, and therefore the time-to-peak concentration is generally not faster than immediate-release carbidopa/levodopa.

  - Occasionally, the immediate-release form is used to make a liquid preparation for PD patients with significant motor fluctuations by mixing 10 tablets of 25/100 mg cabridopa/levodopa with 1/2 teaspoon of ascorbic acid crystals and 1000 mL of distilled water. This preparation allows small and frequent dosing with the goal of relieving wearing off symptoms without causing or worsening peak-dose dyskinesia.

- Abrupt discontinuation of levodopa should be avoided to prevent precipitation of a neuroleptic's malignant-like syndrome characterized by rigidity, hyperthermia, altered consciousness, tachycardia, diaphoresis, and elevated creatine phosphokinase.

- COMT (catechol-O-methyl transferase) inhibitors

  - Entacapone

    - It is a reversible, specific, and mainly peripherally acting catechol-O-methyl transferase (COMT) inhibitor.

    - It decreases the metabolic loss of dopamine to 3-O-methyldopa.

    - It increases the half-life of levodopa by 30–50% so that the levodopa total daily dose may be reduced with no significant effect on the C_{max} (peak concentration) or T_{max} (time to C_{max}).

    - It is particularly indicated for patients experiencing end-of-dose wearing off, but can also be useful in patients with nonfluctuating disease.

    - A single dose of 200 mg to be given together with each dose of levodopa up to eight times daily.

    - There is a small risk of developing diarrhea after 1 month of drug initiation, often requiring drug discontinuation. Entacapone should not be cut in half or chewed as it can discolor teeth yellow-orange. Warn patients also of benign orange discoloration of urine.

  - Stalevo[12]

    - A recently launched combination of entacapone, levodopa, and carbidopa. It comes in three strengths containing 50, 100, and 150 mg of levodopa.

    - Reducing the total daily number of tablets may aid compliance.

  - Tolcapone[13]

    - Another predominantly peripherally acting COMT inhibitor indicated for wearing off symptoms of PD.

    - Available in two doses: 100 mg and 200 mg

    - It has a longer half-life than entacapone and is recommended to be taken no more than three times daily.

- May also cause diarrhea, generally after about 1 month, which often requires discontinuation of the drug.

- Three reported cases of acute liver failure potentially associated with tolcapone use. Therefore, the U.S. Food and Drug Administration requires monthly monitoring of liver function tests for 6 months and as needed thereafter.

- Dopamine agonists

  - Dopamine agonists (DAs) can be used as monotherapy in early disease or as an adjunct in later disease.

  - DAs have a direct action on postsynaptic dopamine receptors.

  - There are several different postsynaptic dopamine receptors: D1, D2, and D3 are the principal subtypes. As DAs vary in their receptor affinity, switching between agents may be clinically advantageous.

  - Five different dopamine agonists are available with varying properties. (Pharmacokinetic properties are summarized in Table 5.5.)

  - When changing from one DA to another, overnight switching may be effective if equivalent doses are used (approximate dose equivalences in a conversion chart are in Table 5.6).

  - Although less potent and subject to more side effects than levodopa, DAs have been proven in several trials to reduce and delay motor fluctuations and delay the need to start levodopa. DAs gonists are, therefore, commonly used early as monotherapy, particularly in younger patients (as they are at higher risk of developing motor fluctuations).

  - DAs can be broadly divided according to the presence of an ergot ring: ergot-based agonists (bromocriptine, pergolide, cabergoline, and lisuride) and nonergot compounds (apomorphine, pramipexole, and ropinirole).

  - Adverse effects of DAs occur as a class effect, with the commonest being nausea, dizziness, ankle swelling, confusion, hallucinations, and psychosis.

    - Adverse effects can be minimized by low initial doses and slow titration. Ropinirole and pergolide have starter packs which ease this process.

TABLE 5.5
Pharmacokinetic Properties of Dopamine Agonists

Preparation	Absorption	Time to max plasma concentration	Bioavailability (%)	Elimination half-life	Clearance
Apomorhine (subcutaneous)	Very rapid	4–12 min	100	33 min	Extrahepatic
Bromocriptine	Rapid	1–3 hr	6	15 hr*	Hepatic
Pergolide	55% absorbed	1–3 hr	20–60	27 hr	Hepatic
Pramipexole	Rapid	1–3 hr	90	8–12 hr‡	Renal
Ropinirole	Rapid	1.5 hr	50	6 hr	Hepatic

* Bromocriptine plasma elimination half life is 3–4 hours for the parent drug and 50 hours for the inactive metabolites. The elimination of parent drug from plasma occurs biphasically, with a terminal half-life of about 15 hours.
‡ 8 hours in the young to 12 hours in the elderly.

TABLE 5.6
Approximate Dose Equivalents for Dopamine Agonists

Bromocriptine (mg tid)	Pergolide (mg tid)	Pramipexole (mg tid)	Ropinirole (mg tid)
1	0.125	0.125	Starter pack then 1 mg tid
2.5	0.25	0.25	1
5	0.5	0.5	2
7.5	0.75	0.75	3
10	1	1	4
12.5	1.25	1.25	6
15	1.5	1.5	8

- Idiosyncratic side effects reported more commonly with dopamine agonists then other PD medications may include: weight gain, compulsive behavior, hypersexuality, and compulsive gambling. Dopamine agonists have also been associated with excessive or sudden-onset sleepiness. Therefore, patients should be counseled about driving, especially during the initiation phase.

- Ergot adverse effects include pulmonary, pericardial, and retroperitoneal fibrosis and have been reported for each of the ergot-based agonists (bromocriptine, pergolide, and cabergoline).

- Subclinical fibrotic heart valve changes detected on echocardiography (particularly the tricuspid valve) have been reported in patients treated with pergolide, but background rates are not clearly defined. Monitoring of symptoms (in particular breathlessness), blood tests (erythrocyte sedimentation rate [ESR] and creatinine), chest x-ray, pulmonary function tests, and echocardiogram are recommended for patients taking these preparations long term.

- Several new dopamine agonist products are under test, including the transdermal agent rotigotine,[14] and controlled-release ropinirole, both of which may reduce fluctuations by long duration of action.

- Apomorphine is a dopamine agonist which undergoes extensive first-pass metabolism and has to be administered parenterally. It is given as bolus sub-cutaneous injections as needed as a "rescue" therapy for wearing off. Currently, it is reserved for patients with advanced disease and significant motor fluctuations. Efficacy is often felt within 10–20 minutes but lasts usually only for 1–1.5 hours. An extended outpatient titration visit if often required to determine the optimal tolerated dose. Premedication with trimethobenzamide 3–7 days prior to initiation is required to minimize gastrointestinal side effects.

- Monoamine oxidase inhibitors
  - Selegiline
    - MAOB inhibitors (MAOBIs) prevent the breakdown of dopamine in the brain and inhibit the reuptake of dopamine at the presynaptic receptor.

    - Enzyme inhibition is irreversible, and therefore activity resumes only after new enzyme has been formed.

    - MAOBIs can be used as an early monotherapy and can prolong the time before levodopa is needed by approximately 9 months.

    - In later disease, adjunctive MAOBI therapy can alleviate dose-related fluctuations and end of dose deterioration.

- The initial interpretation of selegiline studies was of some neuroprotection, but this failed to take account of symptomatic benefits.

- Selegiline is relatively inexpensive.

- Zydis selegiline (Zelapar)

  - Zydis selegiline is a once-daily rapidly dissolving, under-the-tongue freeze-dried tablet formulation of selegiline that was recently approved by the U.S. Food and Drug Administration (FDA) as adjunctive therapy for PD.

  - Dissolves on contact with saliva, eliminating the need for water to aid in swallowing, which can be particularly useful in PD patients who often suffer from dysphagia.

  - As a buccal administration, the tablet undergoes pregastric absorption, minimizing first-pass metabolism and producing high plasma concentrations of selegiline, with a 3- to 10-fold reduction in amphetamine metabolites.

  - A randomized, multicenter, double-blind, 12-week clinical trial evaluated the safety and efficacy of Zydis selegiline[15] (1.25 mg, titrated to 2.5 mg daily, n = 94) versus placebo (n = 46) as adjunctive therapy in PD patients who were experiencing motor fluctuations with L-dopa/carbidopa showed a significant reduction in percentage of off time among patients treated with Zydis selegiline at both weeks 4–6 (with the 1.25 mg dose) (P = .003) and weeks 10–12 (after titration to the 2.5 mg dose) (P <.001). The total number of off hours was reduced by 2.2 hours per day in Zydis selegiline–treated patients compared with 0.6 hours per day in placebo-treated patients (P <.001).

  - It has not been evaluated in head-to-head studies with other adjunct PD therapies or as monotherapy in PD.

- Rasagiline

  - Rasagiline is a selective, second-generation, irreversible MAOBI, with at least five times the potency of selegiline in vitro and in animal models.

- Rasagiline has demonstrated efficacy in one large, randomized double-blind, placebo-controlled trial as initial monotherapy in patients with early PD, and in two large, controlled trials as adjunctive treatment in levodopa-treated PD patients with motor fluctuations.[16–18]

- Unlike selegiline, rasagiline is an aminoindan derivative with no amphetamine metabolites. A randomized clinical trial is underway to confirm preclinical and preliminary clinical data suggesting rasagiline has disease-modifying effects.

- It is available in two doses: 0.5 and 1.0 mg and is to be taken once per day.

- Anticholinergics

  - The use of anticholinergics in PD has declined in recent years due to adverse effects on cognition and the introduction of better alternative dopamine-sparing agents.

  - Structurally related to atropine, these drugs block muscarinic receptors in the striatum, and inhibit the presynaptic carrier-mediated dopamine transport mechanism.

  - Anticholinergics reduce tremor and rigidity, but have little effect on bradykinesia.

  - They may be useful in reducing sialorrhea.

  - They can be used in drug-induced parkinsonism (e.g., in patients taking antipsychotic medication) if the offending drug cannot be withdrawn.

- Amantadine

  - Amantadine is a glutamate antagonist originally developed as an antiviral agent.

  - It enhances dopaminergic transmission and has mild antimuscarinic activity.

  - It has modest antiparkinson effects with a mild improvement in bradykinesia, tremor, and rigidity.

  - Its main use is in more advanced disease, as an antidyskinesia agent.

- ■ Adverse effects include confusion, hallucinations, nervousness, poor concentration, peripheral edema, and livedo reticularis.

- ■ Uusually started at 100 mg twice per day with a top recommended dose of 200 mg twice per day.

■ See Table 5.7 for types of treatments for motor fluctuations.

TABLE 5.7
Treatment of Motor Fluctuations[19]

Motor fluctuation	Established treatments	Other treatment considerations	Experimental approaches
Wearing off	Increase frequency and/or dose of levodopa administration Add dopamine agonist Controlled-release levodopa Add COMT inhibitor Add MAOI Add amantadine	Dietary manipulation Rasagiline Orally disintegrating selegiline	Istradefylline Rotigotine patch
On-off fluctuations	Apomorphine Surgery	Surgery	Duodenal levodopa
Dose Failures	Apomorphine	Improve gastric emptying	Liquid levodopa
Freezing	Levodopa Physical therapy Visual cues	MAOB inhibitors (selegiline, rasagiline) Dopamine agonists	Botulinum toxin
Off period dystonia	Levodopa	Clozapine Botulinum toxin	
Levodopa-induced dyskinesia	Decrease dosage of levodopa Add dopamine agonist while decreasing levodopa Aamantadine Surgery	Clozapine	Talampanel Sarizotan Quetiapine Mementine Remacemide Dextromethorphan Bupidine Idazoxan Liveteracetam Topiramate

Nonmotor Aspects of Parkinsonian Conditions

Cognitive Impairment

- General treatment

    - General approaches to treating the consequences of established dementia in PD follow the same principles applied to other geriatric populations and other dementing illnesses.

    - Infections, metabolic and endocrine derangements, hypoperfusion states, and social stress are also common precipitating factors for worsened mental status and should be addressed or recognized.

    - Substance abuse, including reliance on over-the-counter preparations containing antihistamines, may be underappreciated, especially in individuals who are living alone.

    - Medications with central nervous system (CNS) effects such as narcotics, sedative hypnotics, antidepressants, anxiolytics, and antihistamines should be avoided, or used sparingly.

    - Many other commonly prescribed medications, including antiemetics, antispasmodics for the bladder, H_2 receptor antagonists, antiarrhythmic agents, antihypertensive agents, and nonsteroidal anti-inflammatory agents, may also cause cognitive impairment.

- Specific treatments[20]

    - Cholinesterase inhibitors

        - Four members of this class of compounds are currently FDA approved for the treatment of mild to moderate Alzheimer's disease (AD). Rivastigmine is now also licensed (in the United States and Europe) for treatment of dementia associated with PD.[20]

        - Tacrine, donepezil, rivastigmine, and galantamine are all inhibitors of acetylcholinesterase (AChE) enzyme and, in theory, help repair brain cholinergic deficits by increasing the amount of acetylcholine available for binding in the synaptic cleft to cholinergic receptors.

        - The pharmacokinetic properties and in vivo ability to modulate cholinergic networks of each of these compounds are quite different (Table 5.8).

TABLE 5.8
Cholinesterase Inhibitors FDA-Approved for the Treatment of
Alzheimer's Disease

	Tacrine	Donepezil	Rivastigmine*	Galantamine
Cholinesterase inhibition	Noncompetitive reversible	Noncompetitive reversible	Noncompetitive reversible; most potent	Competitive reversible; least potent
Butryl cholinesterase	+	Negligible	+	Negligible
Nicotinic acetylcholine receptor inhibition	−	−	−	Allosteric modulation
Metabolism	Hepatic CYP450	Hepatic CYP450	Renal	Hepatic, renal
Plasma T1/2	2–4 hr	~70 hr	~1 hr; enzyme dissociation time 8 hr	~6 hr
Dosing	qid	Once daily	bid	bid
Initial dose	5 mg	2.5 mg	1.5 mg	4 mg
Maximum dose	160 mg	10 mg	12 mg	32 mg
Warning label	Hepatotoxicity	−	−	−
Drug interactions	+	+	None known	+

*Also approved for the treatment of Parkinson's dementia.

- For all the cholinesterase inhibitors, the most common side effects are gastrointestinal distress (nausea, diarrhea, vomiting), fatigue, insomnia, and muscle cramps.

- Other strategies

  - Recently, memantine, a noncompetitive antagonist of the NMDA receptor, was approved in the United States as therapy for the treatment of moderate to severe Alzheimer's disease.

  - While there have been few reports showing memantine improves motor symptoms of PD, it has not been yet been reported to improve PD dementia in a double-blind, placebo-controlled trial.

Psychiatric Complications

Psychotic symptoms are common in patients suffering from PD.

■ General treatment

■ As in any geriatric and/or neurologic patient, urinary and pulmonary infections, metabolic and endocrine derangements, cerebral hypoperfusion states, and even social stressors such as changes in the environment are potential precipitating factors for delirium and psychosis in PD. A search for these correctable causes is always required.

■ Another easily ignored etiology is the addition of medications with CNS effects such as narcotics, hypnotics, antidepressants, anxiolytics, and any pharmacologic agent that crosses the blood-brain barrier, including anti-PD medications.

■ If psychotic symptoms persist despite the withdrawal of psychotropic medications, anti-PD medications are then gradually reduced or, if possible, discontinued.

■ Most authorities slowly "peel off" anti-PD drugs in the following order (Figure 5.2).

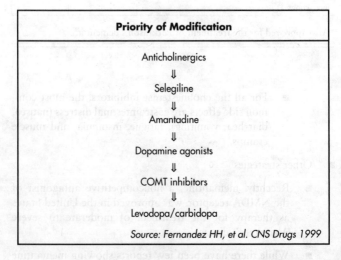

Priority of Modification

Anticholinergics
⇓
Selegiline
⇓
Amantadine
⇓
Dopamine agonists
⇓
COMT inhibitors
⇓
Levodopa/carbidopa

Source: Fernandez HH, et al. CNS Drugs 1999

FIGURE 5.2
Order of anti-PD drug discontinuation in the setting of
drug-induced psychosis.

- Often, reliance on the regular/short-acting formulation of levodopa is preferred over the sustained-release formulation because its pharmacokinetics are more predictable and the shorter half-life means less potential for the cumulative side effects of repeated dosing.

- If psychosis improves, the patient is then maintained on the lowest possible dose of anti-PD medications. However, withdrawal of anti-PD drugs usually worsens parkinsonism and may not be tolerated.

- Atypical antipsychotic (AA) agents[20]:

  - The choice of an AA agent is based largely on its ease of use and side effect profile as most antipsychotic reports, with few exceptions, have comparable efficacy in improving psychosis.

  - The main difference in the antipsychotic agents lies in their propensity to worsen motor functioning in this frail and already vulnerable population.

  - Thus far, six drugs have been marketed in the United States and Europe as "atypical" AA agents: clozapine, risperidone, olanzapine, quetiapine, ziprasidone, and aripiprazole.

  - The use of an AA agent may allow the clinician to control psychosis with fewer motor side effects and, in some cases, without the need for cutting back on anti-PD medications.

    - *Clozapine.* The cumulative experience of all open-label reports on clozapine in parkinsonism involving over 400 patients has been surprisingly consistent. Low doses are required (average of 25 mg/day).

      - A meta-analysis of all large clozapine reports on psychosis in PD showed an 85% improvement rate with acceptable tolerance. Most importantly, clozapine did not worsen motor symptoms. In some reports, it improved tremor.

      - Clozapine remains difficult to use because of its potential for inducing agranulocytosis. The problem is idiosyncratic, so that even the small doses used in PD do not exempt patients from this side effect.

      - In the United States, for the first 6 months, each patient on clozapine undergoes a weekly white blood cell (WBC) count, verified by the pharmacy, and can receive only 1 week's supply of the drug at a time. After 6 months, the process becomes biweekly.

- *Risperidone*. It causes dose-related problems typical of conventional neuroleptics such as prolactin elevation and acute dystonic reactions.

    - Almost all reports concerning risperidone in PD have involved open-label studies.

    - Unfortunately, the studies showed mixed results. A meta-analysis of 82 PD patients treated with risperidone revealed that 23 (33%) experienced motor worsening.

- *Olanzapine*. It is a thiobenzodiazepine of similar chemical structure to clozapine. However, the 2002 Movement Disorders Society Task Force on evidence-based review on the treatment of psychosis in PD concluded that there is "insufficient evidence to demonstrate efficacy of olanzapine in drug-induced psychosis, and it carries an 'unacceptable risk of motor deterioration' even at low conventional doses" based on a disappointing double-blind trial result on PD patients with hallucinations.

- *Quetiapine*. It is a dibenzothiazepine with the closest pharmacologic resemblance to clozapine but without the risk of agranulocytosis.

    - Unfortunately, quetiapine has been subject to only one small, single-center double-blinded trial. Owing to the lack of double-blinded trials, the 2002 Movement Disorder Society Task Force resolved that there is insufficient evidence to conclude on the efficacy or safety of quetiapine in treating drug-induced psychosis in patients with PD.

    - However, several open-label reports involving over 200 PD patients give a fairly solid positive impression on the drug's standing as an atypical antipsychotic agent.

    - Quetiapine appears to be slightly less effective than clozapine against psychosis. Unlike clozapine, it does not improve tremor, and may induce mild motor worsening. But, unlike olanzapine and risperidone, no reported motor worsening with quetiapine has precipitated hospitalization.

- The mean daily dose was generally below 75 mg/d.

- *Ziprasidone.* It was the fifth marketed antipsychotic in the United States with a higher affinity for 5HT2 than D2 receptors. There has been no report on its use in the PD population. A panel of expert psychiatrists reviewing all available data on ziprasidone use in schizophrenia concluded that its extrapyramidal side effect (EPS) profile is "better than risperidone, the same as olanzapine, but not quite as good as quetiapine or clozapine."

- *Aripiprazole.* It is the latest AA drug to be marketed in the United States. This drug is the only AA that is a partial agonist at the D2 and 5HT1a receptors and an antagonist at 5HT2a receptors. It also has a high 5HT2/D2 ratio and may therefore carry a low risk of extrapyramidal side effects while effectively alleviating psychosis in Parkinson-vulnerable populations.

  - The preliminary experience with aripiprazole, however, is mixed but not very encouraging.

- Other agents and treatments:

  - Ondansetron

  - Because of possible antipsychotic effects of $5HT_3$ blockade, ondansetron was tested for treatment of schizophrenia, but has not been found effective.

  - In an open-label trial with 16 PD patients, marked improvement in the areas of visual hallucinations, confusion, and functional impairment was found with no effect on UPDRS scores. Only one patient showed no improvement. However, these positive findings have not been universally reproduced.

  - Acetylcholinesterase (AChE) inhibitors

  - Given the substantial loss of cholinergic neurons in PD, AChE inhibitors might prove useful in PD as well.

  - Several studies on AChE for the treatment of dementia in PD have shown concommitant improvement in hallucinations and other behavioral dysfunctions as well.[20]

- Electroconvulsive therapy

  - ECT is most commonly used for treatment-resistant psychiatric disorders.

  - It has also been reported to improve motor symptoms of PD. In general, ECT's effects are short-lived, and repeated treatments and/or pharmacologic augmentation are required to maintain any benefits.

  - ECT has not been extensively studied in PD-related psychosis.

  - It should probably be reserved for patients who are unresponsive to, or intolerant of, other treatments, especially if psychosis is associated with severe depression.

Behavioral Dysfunction

Depression

- Depressive symptoms may occur at any stage of PD, and is a major factor related to poor quality of life for both the patient and their caregiver.

- It may precede or occur along with or after the onset of motor symptoms.

- There are only a few randomized clinical trials assessing the efficacy and safety of antidepressants in PD.[21]

  - Amitryptyline, desipramine, and nortriptyline all demonstrate antidepressive effects in PD.

  - In three randomized trials comparing tricyclic antidepressants (TCAs) and selective serotonin reuptake inhibitors (SSRIs) in depressed PD patients, amitriptyline was superior in one trial and fluoxetine or sertraline was equally efficacious to amitriptyline in the two other trials.

  - Mirtazapine was superior to placebo in 20 depressed PD patients. Sedation was found to be inversely correlated with dosage. Mirtazapine may possibly improve tremor or dyskinesias.

  - Nefazodone was similar to fluoxetine in improving depression.

- SSRIs and TCAs may be the most useful drugs for the treatment of depression in PD, but SSRIs may be better tolerated (Table 5.9).

- Amoxapine and lithium can cause or worsen parkinsonism and should be avoided in this population.

- Nonselective MAOIs such as isocarboxazid, phenelzine, and tranylcypromine should also be avoided in levodopa-treated patients because of the risk of hypertensive crisis.

- Sedating TCAs (amitriptyline and doxepin) may be beneficial in PD patients with insomnia.

- Tertiary amine TCAs (amitriptyline, doxepin, and imipramine) may be beneficial in PD patients with concomitant bladder hyperactivity and drooling, but harmful in patients with confusion, hallucinations, hypotension, and excessive daytime sleepiness.

- All SSRIs (citalopram, escialopram, fluoxetine, fluvoxamine, paroxetine, sertraline, bupropion [a dopamine agonist reuptake inhibitor], venlafaxine [inhibits 5-HT and norepinephrine reuptake], nefazodone [with antidepressive and anxiolytic properties]) have all been described in PD.

- Electroconvulsive therapy is effective in improving depressive symptoms and transiently improving motor symptoms as well.

- It remains unclear if repetitive transcranial magnetic stimulation also improves depressive and motor symptoms of PD.

Anxiety

- The key to successful management of anxiety in PD is its early recognition. Once anxiety is identified, a team approach to treatment is most beneficial.

  - Nonpharmacologic management that includes education, counseling, and stress-reduction strategies should be an integral part of management of any neurobehavioral disorder.

  - Studies on the pharmacologic management of anxiety in PD are wanting. PD motor symptoms need to be adequately treated. Although most studies find no correlation between PD disability and incidence of anxiety, for

TABLE 5.9
Side Effects of Antidepressants Used in PD

Drug	Dose (mg/d)	Sedation	Hypotension	Antimuscarinic effects	Sexual dysfunction	Weight gain
Fluoxetine	10–80	Negligible	Negligible	Negligible	Considerable	Mild
Fluvoxamine	50–300	Negligible	Negligible	Negligible	Moderate	Moderate
Paroxetine	20–50	Mild	Negligible	Mild	Severe	Moderate
Sertraline	25–100	Negligible	Negligible	Negligible	Moderate	Mild
Citalopram	10–60	Mild	Negligible	Mild	Moderate	Mild
Escitalopram	10–20	Mild	Negligible	Mild	Moderate	Mild
Amitriptyline	25–200	Considerable	Moderate	Considerable	Mild	Considerable
Doxepine	75–150	Moderate	Moderate	Considerable	Mild	Moderate
Imipramine	50–200	Moderate	Considerable	Moderate	Mild	Moderate
Desipramine	100–300	Mild	Mild	Mild	Negligible	Mild
Nortriptyline	50–150	Mild	Mild	Mild	Negligible	Mild
Buproprion	150–450	Negligible	Negligible	Mild	Negligible	Negligible
Mirtazepine	15–45	Moderate	Moderate	Mild	Moderate	Considerable
Nefazodone	300–600	Moderate	Moderate	Negligible	Mild	Negligible
Venlafaxine	75–375	Mild	Negligible	Mild	Considerable	Mild

the subset of patients with motor fluctuations, there is a clear correlation of anxiety with the off states.

■ The majority of PD patients with anxiety will require anxiolytic therapy in addition to dopaminergic medications. There is no adverse interaction between benzodiazepines and dopaminergic therapy, but the potential additive sedative effect of both agents can lead to escalation of daytime somnolence, disruption of sleep-wake cycle, and falling. Cognitively impaired patients can have worsening of their cognition and are at risk for hallucinations. These agents should be avoided in the elderly.

■ SSRIs are becoming the preferred agents for management of essentially any type of anxiety. SSRIs have a favorable side effect profile and limited drug-drug interaction.

■ Concomitant use of SSRIs and MAOIs can lead to the development of serotonin syndrome (SS). Nonselective MAOIs are contraindicated in patients taking levodopa because of the risk of hypertensive crisis. Selegiline does not have a monamine oxidase A (MAOA) inhibitory effect in the prescribed doses below 10 mg/day. However, at higher doses, it becomes a nonselective MAOI. The selegiline and rasagiline package inserts have a warning against the concomitant use of either TCAs or SSRIs owing to the potential central nervous system toxicity such as SS, presenting with alterations of mental status and motor and autonomic dysfunction. Despite the theoretical concern for increased risk of SS with concomitant use of selegiline and antidepressants, it is a rare phenomenon.

■ TCAs act by blocking norepinephrine (noradrenaline) and serotonin uptake as well as producing long-term increase in their receptor sensitivity. There is a role for TCAs in management of PD-related pain and sleep dysfunction, as well as hypersalivation. However, its use in PD is limited by its anticholinergic side effects. TCAs carry a high risk of causing or worsening confusion.

■ Bupropion is a monocyclic antidepressant with indirect dopamine agonist properties. Bupropion improves depression in some PD patients, and may also have a positive effect on PD motor symptoms. The most concerning side effect of the drug is seizures. The effect of bupropion on PD anxiety has not been systematically evaluated but its overall "stimulating" properties may limit its use.

- Buspirone, which pharmacologically is related to bupropion, also has dopamine agonist properties. It can be effective for generalized anxiety disorder, but is less likely to help panic or social phobia.

- Mirtazapine is a newer antidepressant which acts via indirect enhancement of serotonin 5-HT1 receptors as well as direct inhibition of alpha$_2$ presynaptic adrenergic receptors. It has been shown to be effective in generalized anxiety disorder.

Pathologic Gambling and Punding

- There are two types of OCD-like behaviors recently described in PD:

1. Pathologic gambling is classified under *impulse control disorders* in the DSM-IV and is characterized by "failure to resist the impulse to gamble despite personal, family or vocational consequences." In most reports, the behavior appears after the onset of PD,[22] more often in the on state, and is more closely associated with dopamine agonists than with levodopa. It resolves with atypical antipsychotic agents or cessation of anti-PD medications.

2. Punding[23] was first observed among amphetamine and cocaine abusers but has now been described in PD as well. It is a stereotypical motor behavior in which there is an intense fascination with repetitive handling and examining of mechanical objects, such as picking at one-self or taking apart watches and radios or sorting and arranging of common objects, such as lining up pebbles or rocks. Although punding may be considered a form of compulsion, the actions are not usually perceived by the patient as relieving a sense of inner tension as is usually the case in OCD. It usually occurs after chronic dopaminergic therapy and is relieved by reduction of anti-PD medications.

Sleep Disturbances

- Sleep complaints have been reported in over 60% of PD patients (Table 5.10).[24,25]

TABLE 5.10
Spectrum of Sleep Disturbances in PD

Disorders of sleep initiation and maintenance	Insomnia
Parasomnias	Sleep fragmentation (frequent nighttime awakenings)
	Early arousal
	Periodic leg movements of sleep
	Restless legs syndrome
	Obstructive sleep apnea
	REM sleep behavior disorder (RBD)
	Nocturnal vocalizations
	Somnambulism
	Nightmares
	Night terrors
Excessive daytime sleepiness	Medication effect
	Sudden onset sleep
	DBS surgery effect
Cognitive-behavioral dysfunction contributing to sleep dysfunction	Depression
	Anxiety
	Visual hallucinations
	Dementia

REM, rapid eye movement.

Management

■ Good sleep hygiene with regular sleep-wake hours and regular meal times.

■ Dopaminergic therapy may need to be reduced if nocturnal dyskinesias are present; increased if nocturnal akinesia is predominant.

■ Controlled-release levodopa may provide added benefit for patients with nocturnal akinesia and early morning worsening of symptoms.

■ Recognition and treatment of related disorders such as depression, anxiety, and psychosis.

- For excessive daytime sleepiness or sudden-onset sleep, avoiding or reducing the offending agent (such as dopamine agonists) or adding modafinil, methylphenidate, caffeine, dextroamphetamine, or other similar agents.

- For restless legs syndrome, dopamine agonists, controlled-release levodopa, gabapentin, clonazepam, and opiates are potential treatments.

- For periodic limb movements during sleep and rapid eye movement (REM) behavior disorder, low-dose clonazepam is usually helpful.

Autonomic Dysfunction

- Over the course of PD, more than 90% of patients experience symptoms of autonomic dysfunction, which often results in a negative impact on quality of life (Tables 5.11 and 5.12).[26]

TABLE 5.11
Nonpharmacologic Treatments of Autonomic Dysfunction in PD

Symptom	Treatment options
Orthostatic hypotension	Taper or discontinue unnecessary hypotensive drugs
	Elevate head of bed 10–30 degrees
	Increase dietary salt (add salt tablets)
	Thigh-high, fitted compression stockings
	Education: for example, avoid standing quickly, hot environment, straining-type exercises
Dysphagia	Double swallowing, using a "chin tuck"
	Increase consistency of food
	Adjust timing of medications (e.g., 20–30 minutes before meals)
	Feeding tube placement
Constipation	Add dietary bulk
	Increase fluid intake
	Regular exercise
Excessive drooling	Encourage voluntary swallowing of saliva
	Sugar-free gum or hard candy

TABLE 5.12
Pharmacologic Options for Autonomic Dysfunction in PD

Symptom	Drug	Dose
Orthostatic hypotension	Fludrocortisone	0.1 mg daily
	Midodrine	5–10 mg tid; last dose should not be after 6 PM to avoid supine hypertension
	Ephedrine	25–50 mg q4–6 hr
	Phenylpropanolamine	
	Ergotamine/caffeine	
	May consider: physostigmine, erythropoietin, or octreotide	
Constipation	Stool softeners (e.g., docusate sodium)	50–200 mg daily PO
	Osmotic laxatives (lactulose, milk of magnesia)	15–30 mL lactulose daily PO
	Stimulant laxative (bisacodyl)	10–15 mg PO once daily; 10 mg per rectum once daily; or 30 mL Fleet enema
	Mineral/tap water enemas	
Excessive drooling	Trihexyphenidyl	2.0–5.0 mg tid
	Benztropine	0.5–1.0 mg tid
	glycopyrrolate	1.0–2.0 mg tid/qid
	Botulinum toxin type A or B	Injection into parotid and salivary gland
Erectile dysfunction	Sildenafil	50–100 mg 1 hr prior to intercourse; watch for orthostatic hypotension
	Vardenafil	5–20 mg 1 hr prior to intercourse
	Tadalafil	5–20 mg 1 hr prior to intercourse
	Yohimbine	5 mg tid
	Papaverine	Intracavernous injection
Urinary frequency (hyperactive bladder)	Tolterodine	2 mg bid
	Oxybutynin	5 mg tid/qid; patch q3 days

continued

TABLE 5.12 (cont.)

Symptom	Drug	Dose
	Propantheline	15–30 mg qid
	Hyoscyamine	0.15–0.3 mg qhs–qid
	Imipramine	10–25 mg at bedtime
Urinary retention (hypoactive bladder)	Terazosin	
	Doxazosin	1–4 mg daily
	Prazosin	1 mg bid–tid; may increase slowly up to 20 mg/day
	Tamsulosin	0.4–0.8 mg daily
	Bethanechol chloride	10–50 mg PO tid–qid; 2.5–5 mg SC tid–qid
Pain	Minimize off time	Increasing/optimizing dopaminergic medications
	Consider apomorphine	2–10 mg SC with each off state; not more than 10 injections per day

REFERENCES

1. Frigerio R, Elbaz A, Sanft KR et al. Education and occupations preceding Parkinson disease: a population-based case-control study. Neurology 2005;65(10):1575–1583.
2. de Lau LM, Breteler MM. Epidemiology of Parkinson's disease. Lancet Neurol 2006;5(6):525–535.
3. Hughes AJ, Daniel SE, Kilford L, Lees AJ. Accuracy of clinical diagnosis of idiopathic Parkinson's disease: a clinico-pathological study of 100 cases. J Neurol Neurosurg Psychiatry 1992;55(3):181–184.
4. Fujimoto K. Vascular parkinsonism. J Neurol 2006;253(Suppl 3): iii16–iii21.
5. Kowalska A, Jamrozik Z, Kwiecinski H. Progressive supranuclear palsy—parkinsonian disorder with tau pathology. Folia Neuropathol 2004;42(2):119–123.
6. Uchihara T, Mitani K, Mori H et al. Abnormal cytoskeletal pathology peculiar to corticobasal degeneration is different from that of Alzheimer's disease or progressive supranuclear palsy. Acta Neuropathol (Berl) 1994;88(4):379–383.
7. Feany MB, Dickson DW. Widespread cytoskeletal pathology characterizes corticobasal degeneration. Am J Pathol 1995;146(6): 1388–1396.
8. Walshe JM. Hepatic Wilson's disease: initial treatment and long-term management. Curr Treat Options Gastroenterol 2005;8(6):467–472.

9. Marmarou A, Young HF, Aygok GA et al. Diagnosis and management of idiopathic normal-pressure hydrocephalus: a prospective study in 151 patients. J Neurosurg 2005;102(6):987–997.

10. Zesiewicz TA, Elble R, Louis ED et al. Practice parameter: therapies for essential tremor: report of the Quality Standards Subcommittee of the American Academy of Neurology. Neurology 2005; 64(12):2008–2020.

11. Hubble JP, Busenbark KL, Wilkinson S et al. Deep brain stimulation for essential tremor. Neurology 1996;46(4):115–1103.

12. Koller W, Guarnieri M, Hubble J et al. An open-label evaluation of the tolerability and safety of Stalevo (carbidopa, levodopa and entacapone) in Parkinson's disease patients experiencing wearing-off. J Neural Transm 2005;112(2):221–230.

13. Kurth MC, Adler CH, Hilaire MS et al. Tolcapone improves motor function and reduces levodopa requirement in patients with Parkinson's disease experiencing motor fluctuations: a multicenter, double-blind, randomized, placebo-controlled trial. Tolcapone Fluctuator Study Group I. Neurology 1997;48(1):817.

14. Poewe W, Luessi F. Clinical studies with transdermal rotigotine in early Parkinson's disease. Neurology 2005;65(2 Suppl 1):S114.

15. Waters CH, Sethi KD, Hauser RA et al. Zydis selegiline reduces off time in Parkinson's disease patients with motor fluctuations: a 3-month, randomized, placebo-controlled study. Mov Disord 2004;19(4):426–432.

16. Rabey JM, Sagi I, Huberman M et al. Rasagiline mesylate, a new MAO-B inhibitor for the treatment of Parkinson's disease: a double-blind study as adjunctive therapy to levodopa. Clin Neuropharmacol 2000;23(6):324–330.

17. Rascol O, Brooks DJ, Melamed E et al. Rasagiline as an adjunct to levodopa in patients with Parkinson's disease and motor fluctuations (LARGO, Lasting effect in Adjunct therapy with Rasagiline Given Once daily, study): a randomised, double-blind, parallel-group trial. Lancet 2005;365(9463):947–954.

18. Stern MB, Marek KL, Friedman J et al. Double-blind, randomized, controlled trial of rasagiline as monotherapy in early Parkinson's disease patients. Mov Disord 2004;19(8):916–923.

19. Pahwa R, Factor SA, Lyons KE et al. Practice parameter: treatment of Parkinson disease with motor fluctuations and dyskinesia (an evidence-based review): report of the Quality Standards Subcommittee of the American Academy of Neurology. Neurology 2006; 66(7):983–995.

20. Poewe W, Wolters E, Emre M et al. Long-term benefits of rivastigmine in dementia associated with Parkinson's disease: an active treatment extension study. Mov Disord 2006;21(4):456–461.

21. Miyasaki JM, Shannon K, Voon V et al. Practice parameter: evaluation and treatment of depression, psychosis, and dementia in Parkinson disease (an evidence-based review): report of the Quality Standards Subcommittee of the American Academy of Neurology. Neurology 2006;66(7):996–1002.

22. Stocchi F. Pathological gambling in Parkinson's disease. Lancet Neurol 2005;4(10):590–592.

23. Voon V. Repetition, repetition, and repetition: compulsive and punding behaviors in Parkinson's disease. Mov Disord 2004;19(4): 367–370.

24. Adler CH, Thorpy MJ. Sleep issues in Parkinson's disease. Neurology 2005;64(12 Suppl 3):S1220.

25. Gagnon JF, Postuma RB, Mazza S et al. Rapid-eye-movement sleep behaviour disorder and neurodegenerative diseases. Lancet Neurol 2006;5(5):424–432.

26. Korchounov A, Kessler KR, Yakhno NN et al. Determinants of autonomic dysfunction in idiopathic Parkinson's disease. J Neurol 2005;252(12):1530–1536.

6

THE "TWISTED" PATIENT

PHENOMENOLOGY

Dystonia is a neurologic syndrome characterized by involuntary, sustained, patterned, and often repetitive muscle contractions of opposing muscles causing twisting movements or abnormal postures. Partly because of its rich expression and a variable course, dystonia is frequently not recognized or is misdiagnosed."[1]

The prevalence of generalized primary torsion dystonia in Rochester, Minnesota, was reported to be 3.4 per 100,000 population, and focal dystonia as 30 per 100,000 population.[2]

Main Features

- Relatively long duration (unlike chorea or myoclonus in which the involuntary movements are brief).

- Both agonist and antagonist muscles of a body part simultaneously contract, which results in twisting of the affected body part.

- The same muscle groups are generally involved, unlike chorea in which the involuntary movements are random and involve different muscle groups.

Other Features

- Primary dystonia almost always begins by affecting a single part of the body (focal dystonia), which then gradually generalizes; most often the spread is to contiguous body parts.

■ The younger the age at onset, the more likely for dystonia to spread (e.g., childhood onset with leg involvement usually leads to eventual generalized dystonia).[3,4]

■ Dystonia is almost always worsened with voluntary movement. Dystonic movement may be aggravated during voluntary movements and may be termed *action dystonia*. Abnormal dystonic movements that appear only during certain actions are termed *task-specific dystonia*—an example is writer's cramp.

■ As the dystonia progresses, even nonspecific voluntary action can bring out dystonia; eventually actions in other parts of the body can induce dystonic movements of the primarily affected body part, termed *overflow dystonia*.

■ Dystonia usually worsens with fatigue and stress, and is suppressed with sleep, hypnosis, or relaxation.

■ A unique and intriguing feature of dystonia is that the movements can be suppressed by tactile or proprioceptive "sensory tricks" (geste antagoniste): lightly touching the affected body part can often reduce the muscle contractions.

■ Surprisingly, pain is not very common in dystonia except in cervical dystonia, in which up to 75% of patients experienced pain in one study.[5]

■ Dystonia can present with tremor (dystonic tremor) or myoclonus (dystonia-myoclonus). Dystonic tremor from cervical dystonia can be distinguished from essential tremor as the dystonic tremor is usually less regular or rhythmic than essential tremor and is associated with a head tilt and chin deviation.

■ Rarely, children and adolescents with primary or secondary dystonia can develop a sudden and marked increase in the severity of dystonia, termed *dystonic storm*.

CLASSIFICATION

By Distribution

■ *Focal ldystonia* affects a single body part (e.g., torticollis, writer's cramp, blepharospasm, foot dystonia, lingual dystonia, spasmodic dysphonia).

- *Segmental dystonia* affects one or more contiguous body parts (e.g., Meige's syndrome).

- *Multifocal dystonia* involves two or more noncontiguous body parts.

- *Hemidystonia* involves only half the body; usually associated with a structural lesion (e.g., tumor in the contralateral putamen).

- *Generalized dystonia* affects the entire body.

By Clinical Features

Continual

- Primary (or idiopathic) dystonia

  - May be inherited or sporadic.

  - Can be early onset (<26 years old) or late onset (>26 years old)

    - Younger onset dystonias tend to become severe and are more likely to spread to involve multiple parts of the body.

    - Older onset dystonias tend to remain focal.

- Secondary

  - May be generalized, segmental, focal, or multifocal and associated with other neurologic disorders.

  - Unilateral/hemidystonia is often symptomatic, usually resulting from, e.g., a stroke, trauma, arteriovenous malformation (AVM), or tumor.

Fluctuating

- Paroxysmal dyskinesias can vary from chorea/ballism to the sustained contractions of dystonia. *Paroxysmal* is the most common term used for periodic choreoathetotic and dystonic involuntary movements, while *episodic* is most commonly used for periodic ataxic involuntary movements. Paroxysmal dyskinesias are generally classified into three types (Table 6.1):

  - Paroxysmal kinesogenic dyskinesia (PKD)

    - Usually lasts for seconds to minutes; precipitated by sudden movement, startle, or hyperventilation; occurring

TABLE 6.1
Summary of Features of Major Causes of Paroxysmal Dyskinesias

	PKD	PND	PED
Male/female ratio	4:1	3:2	Unclear
Age of onset	5–15	Less than 5 years	2–20
Inheritance	AD, sporadic	AD, sporadic	AD
Duration of attacks	<5 min	Several minutes to hours	5–30 min
Frequency	Very frequent, 100/day to 1/month	Occasional, 3/day to 2/year	1/day to 1/month
Asymmetry	Common	Less common	
Ability to suppress attacks	Able	Able	
Precipitating factors	Sudden movement, startle, hyperventilation, fatigue, stress	Alcohol, caffeine, exercise, excitement	Prolonged exercise, stress, caffeine, fatigue
Associated features	Dystonia, chorea, epilepsy	Chorea, dystonia, ataxia	Dystonia, chorea
Treatment	Phenytoin, carbamazepine, barbiturates, acetazolamide	Clonazepam, oxazepam	

AD, autosomal dominant; PED, paroxysmal exertional dyskinesia; PKD, paroxysmal kinesogenic dyskinesia; PND, paroxysmal nonkinesogenic dyskinesia.

many times a day; patients may experience a sensory aura prior to the attack.

■ The majority of etiologies are primary (familial-autosomal dominant or sporadic); secondary causes of PKD include multiple sclerosis, head injury, hypoxia, hypoparathyroidism, and basal ganglia and thalamic strokes.

■ May respond to anticonvulsants, especially when the duration of paroxysmal attacks is brief.

■ Paroxysmal nonkinesogenic dyskinesia

■ Often consists of any combination of dystonic postures, chorea, athetosis, and ballism; may be unilateral or bilateral; longer duration and smaller frequency of attacks compared to PKD.

- Precipitated by alcohol, coffee, tea, stress, fatigue.

- Etiology could be primary (familial-autosomal dominant or sporadic) or secondary (from, e.g., multiple sclerosis, hypoxia, encephalitis, metabolic causes, psychogenic).

- Not sensitive to anticonvulsants.

- Paroxysmal exertional dyskinesia

  - Attacks are more brief than PKND lasting 5–30 minutes; precipitated by prolonged exercise.

  - Most familial cases follow an autosomal dominant inheritance.

  - May respond to anticonvulsants or antimuscarinics.

- Paroxysmal hypnogenic dyskinesia

  - Can be brief or prolonged attacks.

  - Several cases may be due to supplementary or frontal lobe seizures.

- Diurnal

  - Aromatic acid decarboxylase deficiency (usually in infancy, with axial hypotonia, athetosis, ocular convergence spasm, oculogyric crises, limb rigidity).

  - GTP cyclohydrolase I deficiency (DYT5): first step in tetrahydrobiopterin synthesis; childhood onset, may be diurnal, improves with low-dose levodopa; abnormal phenylalanine loading test.

- Other causes: side effect of levodopa therapy, acute dystonic reactions to neuroleptics, gastroesophageal reflux, oculogyric crisis (sudden, transient conjugate eye deviation).

By Etiology

1. *Primary (idiopathic)*. May be familial (Table 6.2) or sporadic; pure dystonic syndromes.

2. *Dystonia-plus.* "Nonneurodegenerative" conditions in which signs and symptoms other than dystonia such as parkinsonism and myoclonus are present; these are generally not

TABLE 6.2
Genetic Classification of the Dystonias

Type	Chromosome/Gene	Inheritance	Features	Reference no.
DYT1	9q34/torsin A; deletion of one pair of GAG triplets	AD; penetrance rate 30–40%	Young-onset; 1/2000 in the Ashkenazi Jewish population; commercial testing is available; early onset (<26 years old testing is useful); limbs affected first; pure dystonia; MRI normal	6
DYT2		AR	Described in Spanish gypsies	7
DYT3	Xq13.1	X-linked	"Lubag," Filipino males, dystonia-parkinsonism	8
DYT4			"Whispering dysphonia" family	9
DYT5	14q22.1/GTP cyclohydrolase-1	AD	Dopa-responsive dystonia	10
DYT6	8p21-q22	AD	Mixed type; in the Mennonite/Amish populations; childhood and adult-onset; site of onset in arm/cranial > leg/neck; usually remains as upper body	11
DYT7	18p	AD	Adult-onset familial torticollis in a northwestern German family; occasional arm involvement	12
DYT8	2q33-q35	AD	Paroxysmal nonkinesogenic dyskinesia	13,14
DYT9	1p21	AD	Paroxysmal dyskinesia with spasticity	15
DYT10	16p11.2-q12.1	AD	Paroxysmal kinesogenic dyskinesia	16
DYT11	7q21-q23/epsilon-sargoglycan	AD	Myoclonus-dystonia syndrome; alcohol responsive	17
DYT12	19q	AD	Rapid-onset dystonia parkinsonism	18

TABLE 6.2 (cont.)

Type	Chromosome/Gene	Inheritance	Features	Reference no.
DYT13	1p36.13-p36.32	AD	Adult-onset familial cranial-cervical-brachial predominant; site of onset is usually neck; remains segmental	19
DYT14	14q14	AD	Dopamine-responsive dystonia	20
DYT15	18p11	AD	Myoclonus-dystonia syndrome	21

AD = autosomal dominant; AR = autosomal recessive.

neurodegenerative disorders, but would be better classified as neurochemical disorders.

- **Dopa-responsive dystonia (DRD)**

  - GTP cyclohydrolase I deficiency (DYT5): childhood onset (<16 years); females > males; may be diurnal (worse at night); parkinsonism; improves with low-dose levodopa; adult onset with parkinsonism or focal dystonia; abnormal phenylalanine loading test.

  - Autosomal recessive with mutation of tyrosine hydroxylase gene.

  - Other biopterin deficiencies.

  - May be mistaken for juvenile Parkinson's disease (PD) and childhood primary torsion dystonia (Table 6.3).

- **Dopamine agonist–responsive dystonia.** Aromatic acid decarboxylase deficiency; autosomal recessive mode of inheritance.

- **Rapid-onset dystonia parkinsonism (RDP).** Autosomal dominant; chromosome 19q13; adolescent or adult onset; dystonia generalizes over a few days to weeks; with parkinsonism; generally stabilizes within a few weeks with slow or no progression; little or no response to levodopa or dopamine agonists.

- **Myoclonus-dystonia syndrome.** Dystonia with myoclonic jerks that respond to alcohol; autosomal dominant; chromosome 7q21/18p11; upper part of the body affected; childhood,

TABLE 6.3
Features Distinguishing Juvenile Parkinsonism (PD),
Dopa-Responsive Dystonia (DRD), and Childhood Primary
Torsion Dystonia (PTD)

Feature	DRD	Juvenile PD	Childhood PTD
Gender predisposition	Female	Male	None
Dystonia presentation	Dystonia throughout the course, occasionally improves with sleep; starts in the foot or leg; with bradykinesia	Dystonia at the onset, may be diurnal and improves with sleep; starts in the foot; with parkinsonism	Dystonia throughout the course, without diurnal pattern or sleep benefit; no signs of parkinsonism or bradykinesia
Treatment response	Low-dose Sinemet* and anticholinergic drugs	Higher doses of Sinemet*; all other anti-PD agents including anticholinergic drugs	Unlikely to respond to Sinemet* but responds to anticholinergic drugs
Course	Plateaus	Progressive	Usually progressive

*Combination of carbidopa and levopdopa.

adolescent ,or adult onset; slowly progressive and tends to plateau; may be associated with other psychiatric features such as substance abuse, anxiety, psychosis.

3. *Secondary dystonia.* That due to environmental insult (Table 6.4).

4. *Heredodegenerative dystonia.* That due to neurodegenerative diseases; usually inherited; usually not pure dystonia (Table 6.5) (Figure 6.1).

5. A feature of another neurologic disease. For example, tics, paroxysmal dyskinesias, PD, PSP.

6. *Pseudodystonia*

■ Not true dystonia but sustained abnormal postures are present.

■ Examples include stiff person syndrome, Isaacs' syndrome, Satoyoshi's syndrome, chronic inflammatory myopathy,[22]

TABLE 6.4
Symptomatic Causes of Dystonia

Perinatal cerebral injury with kernicterus	Athetoid cerebral palsy, delayed-onset dystonia
Infection	Viral encephalitis Encephalitis lethargica Reye's syndrome Subacute sclerosing panencephalitis Creutzfeldt-Jakob disease HIV infection
Drugs	Levodopa and dopamine agonists Dopamine receptor–blocking agents Fenfluramine Anticonvulsants Flecainide Ergots Some calcium channel blockers
Toxins	Manganese Carbon monoxide Carbon disulfide Cyanide Methanol Disulfiram 3-Nitroproprionic acid Wasp sting toxin
Metabolic	Hypoparathyroidism
Brain/brainstem lesions	Paraneoplastic brainstem encephalitis Primary antiphospholipid syndrome CVA, ischemic injury Central pontine myelinolysis Multiple sclerosis Tumors AVM Trauma Surgery (thalamotomy)
Spinal cord lesions, syringomyelia	
Peripheral lesions	Lumbar stenosis Trauma Electrical injury

AVM, arteriovenous malformation; CVA, cerebrovascular accident.

Sandifer's syndrome, bone disease, ligamentous absence, congenital muscular torticollis (commonly associated with a sternomastoid tumor), juvenile rheumatoid arthritis, seizures.

TABLE 6.5
Heredodegenerative Disorders with Dystonic Manifestations

Inheritance	Disease	Features	Diagnosis
X-linked	Lubag (X-linked dystonia-parkinsonism) (DYT3)	Filipino males living in the Island of Panay; young adult onset; cranial or generalized dystonia; parkinsonism can appear at onset or develop later; progressive, disabling	Clinical; gene test not currently commercially available
	Deafness-dystonia syndrome (Mohr-Tranebjaerg syndrome)	Deafness and dystonia in males	
	Pelizaeus-Merzbacher disease	Deficiency in myelin-specific lipids; partial to total absence of myelination; ataxia, nystagmus, hypotonia; dystonia occurs later and progresses slowly	
	Rett's syndrome	X-linked dominant (therefore occurs only in girls); characteristically combines psychomotor regression, loss of purposeful use of hands and stereotypia, ataxia, and apraxia of gait with microcephaly; dystonia, and oculogyric crises in over 50%	Clinical
Autosomal dominant	Juvenile parkinsonism	May present with dystonia initially (see Table 6.2)	Clinical/genetic
	Huntington's disease	Usually presents with chorea but dystonia is common. Commonly manifesting between ages 30 and 54 but can present at any age. Progressive disorder with varying degrees of cognitive and psychiatric dysfunction	Gene testing, iT15 CAG expansion

TABLE 6.5 (cont.)

Inheritance	Disease	Features	Diagnosis
	Machado-Joseph disease (SCA3)	Mainly affecting families descending from the ancestors in the Portuguese islands of the Azores; dystonia in about 20%; type I: predominantly pyramidal-extrapyramidal signs; type II: cerebellar plus pyramidal; type III: cerebellar plus distal amyotrophy	Genetic, CAG expansion 14q
	Dentatorubropallido-luysian atrophy	Degeneration of cerebellar, efferent, and pallidoluysian systems; dystonia is not usually prominent; adult-onset: ataxia, choreoathetosis, dementia; juvenile-onset: presents like progressive myoclonic epilepsy	Genetic, CAG expansion 21 p
	Other spinocerebellar ataxias	Because phenotypic variability is great, a complete ataxia genetic screening profile is recommended	Genetic
Autosomal recessive	Wilson's disease	Can also present with tremor, dystonia, or parkinsonism; usually below age 50; abnormal metabolism of copper and linked to chromosome 13; damage results in copper accumulation (See Figure 6.1)	Kayser-Fleischer rings; ceruloplasmin gene defects of chromosome 13; liver biopsy
	Niemann-Pick disease type C	Dystonic lipidosis; sea-blue histiocytosis; in type C, there is no specific enzymatic deficit described; sphingomyelinase activity is normal in most tissues; patients with later onset present with characteristic supranuclear gaze palsy, mental decline, gait disorder, ataxia, and dystonia.	Defective cholesterol sterification/ sphingomyelinase

continued

TABLE 6.5 (cont.)

Inheritance	Disease	Features	Diagnosis
	Juvenile neuronal ceroid-lipofuscinosis	Marked by storage of lipopigments; with infantile, late infantile, juvenile, and adult form; juvenile form present without visual failure and with myoclonic epilepsy, dementia, behavioral and extrapyramidal signs, especially facial dyskinesias	Pathology (rectal biopsy)
	GM1 gangliosidosis	GM1 is characterized by visceromegaly, cognitive decline, dysmorphism, an a cherry-red spot in the macular region; types 1, 2, 3 in children; type 3 present 2–27 years of age with variable manifestations including ataxia, dystonia, and myopathy; in adults, GM1 is characterized by dystonia and early-onset parkinsonism with prolonged survival	ß-D-galactosidase deficiency
	GM2 gangliosidosis	Deficiency of lysosomal hexosaminidase; more frequent among Ashkenzi Jews from Eastern Europe; infantile GM2 has an aggressive course with spastic tetraparesis, seizures, and blindness with dystonia later in the course; in juvenile, chronic, and adult GM2, dystonia may be the presenting feature (usually legs)	Hexosaminidase deficiency
	Metachromatic leukodystrophy	Deficiency in cerebroside sulfatase leading to sulfatide accumulation; may present with mental decline, behavioral dysfunction, and dystonia	Aryl sulfatase A deficiency

TABLE 6.5 (cont.)

Inheritance	Disease	Features	Diagnosis
	Lesch-Nyhan syndrome	May present with generalized dystonia; age of onset in children, with mental retardation, self-mutilation, hyperuricemia	Hypoxanthine guanine phosphoribosyl transferase deficiency
	Homocystinuria	May present with generalized dystonia in children; with focal deficits, ectopia lentis, skeletal deformities, and mental retardation; neuroimaging may show focal ischemic lesions, sinus thrombosis	Amino acid chromatog-raphy
	Glutaric acidemia	Along with cerebral palsy, is one of the leading causes of dystonia in the first year of life; generalized dystonia with mental retardation	Glutaric acid in the urine; glutaryl-Co-A dehydrogenase deficiency
	Methylmalonic aciduria	Generalized dystonia in children with acute encephalopathy	Chromatography of organic acids; methylmalonic CoA mutase
	Ataxia-telangiectasia	Generalized dystonia in children with ataxia and neuropathy; cerebellar atrophy on imaging	Clinical; low levels of IgA
	Neurodegeneration with brain iron accumulation; pantothenate kinase–associated neurodegeneration	Formerly called Hallervorden-Spatz syndrome; characterized by iron deposition in the pallidum; dystonia may be associated with tics and other movement disorders	Pathology; imaging showing pallidal T2 hypointensity ("eye of the tiger" sign)

continued

TABLE 6.5 (cont.)

Inheritance	Disease	Features	Diagnosis
	Neuroacanthocytosis	Usually start in the third decade with orobuccolingual hyperkinesia, lip smacking, vocalizations, and even orolingual action dystonia leading to lip and tongue automutilation; 50% with seizures; most with polyneuropathy, distal amyotrophy, pes cavus	Acanthocytes in peripheral smear
Mitochondrial	Leigh's disease	Generalized dystonia in children with hypotonia, ataxia, optic atrophy	Pyruvic acid and alanine levels, mtDNA mutations, cytochrome oxidase activity

- Psychogenic dystonia. The following are clues that suggest psychogenic dystonia:

  - Abrupt onset.

  - Changing characteristics over time.

  - Movements do not fit with known patterns.

  - Accompanied by other types of movements (e.g., rhythmical shaking, bizarre gait, astasia-abasia, excessive startle or slowness).

  - Associated with other features (e.g., false weakness and sensory complaints, psychiatric disorders, secondary gain pending litigation, multiple somatizations).

  - Spontaneous remission.

  - Improvement with distraction.

  - Paroxysmal or intermittent nature.

  - Twisting facial movements (especially side-to-side movements of the mouth).

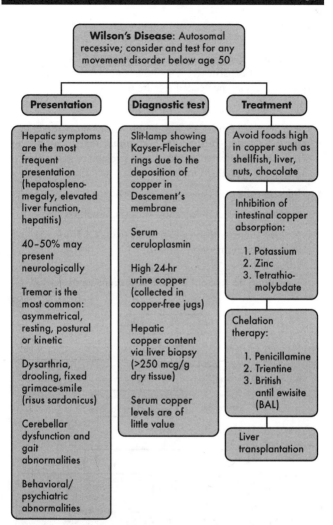

FIGURE 6.1

The presentation, diagnosis, and treatment of Wilson's disease.

TREATMENT

Focus on the etiology of dystonia; management can be difficult; patients do not consistently respond to one type of therapy; multiple strategies may be needed (Figure 6.2).

    1. Oral medications (see Table 6.6).

    2. Chemodenervation: Botulinum toxin—a product of an anaerobic bacteria, *Clostridium botulinum*, that is purified and injected into the affected muscles; two strains are available: type A (Botox) and type B (Myobloc).

■ Injection sites:

    ■ Blepharospasm injection sites (Figure 6.3):

        ■ Start with very low doses (e.g., 2.5 U for type A for each injection site).

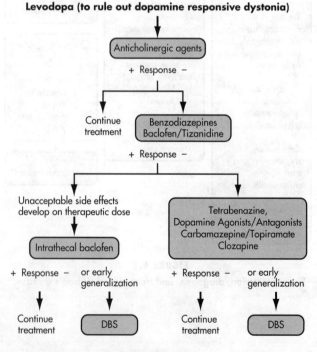

FIGURE 6.2

Treatment algorithm for generalized dystonia. This treatment algorithm is not applicable to dystonia from treatable metabolic disorders. DBS, Deep brain stimulation surgery.

TABLE 6.6
Common Medications Used for the Symptomatic Treatment of Dytonia

Medication	Typical starting dose (mg/d)	Typical therapeutic dose (mg/d)	Comments
Carbidopa/levodopa	25/100	Up to 800	To be given 3 times per day; always try levodopa first, especially if young to rule out DRD—requires only low dose
Trihexyphenidyl	1–2	Up to 120	In divided doses; if increased very slowly, young patients are able to tolerate high doses
Benztropine	0.5–1	Up to 8	Watch for anticholinergic side effects
Baclofen	5–10	Up to 120	GABA agonist; do not abruptly discontinue (risk of seizures)
Clonazepam	0.5–1	Up to 5	
Tetrabenazine	25	Up to 75	Available in Canada, UK
Tizanidine	2	24	Unlike baclofen, minimal risk of seizures with abrupt discontinuation

DRD, dopamine-responsive dystonia.

- Inject the upper orbicularis oculi muscle as close to the eyelid margin for maximum efficacy and the least side effect.

- Avoid the middle upper eyelid area (where the levator palpebrae lies) to prevent ptosis.

- Use a 30-gauge × 1/2-inch needle

- Cervical dystonia (Figure 6.4):

    - Sternocleidomastoid muscle (SCM). Responsible for anterocollis and contralateral chin deviation.

    - Splenius capitis (SPC), Responsible for retrocollis (the most common presentation of tardive dystonia) and ipsilateral chin deviation.

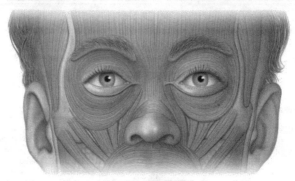

FIGURE 6.3
Blepharospasm: injection sites.

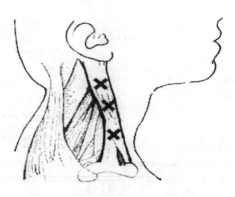

FIGURE 6.4
Cervical dystonia injection sites.

- ■ Trapeziums (TRAP). Responsible for ipsilateral shoulder elevation.

- ■ Levator scapulae (LS).Responsible for ispsilateral shoulder elevation.

- ■ Scalenus complex (SCAL). Responsible for ipsilateral head tilt.

- ■ Submentalis (SM). Responsible for anterocollis.

■ Usual doses (Table 6.7):

  - ■ Botox (comes in 100 U/vial powdered form to be diluted with preservative-free normal saline).

TABLE 6.7
Typical Doses of Botulinum Toxin Type A (Botox) and B (Myobloc)

Presentation	Muscle	Average starting dose (Botox) (U)	Average dose (Botox) (U)	Starting Dose Range (Myobloc) (U)
Blepharospasm	Orbicularis oculi	2.5–5/site	5–10/site	250–000/site
	Procerus	2.5–5/site	2.5–10/site	250–500
Hemifacial spasm*	Orbicularis oris	2.5/site	2.5–5/site	125–750
	Levator anguli oris	2.5–10	2.5–10	125–250
	Depressor anguli oris	2.5–10	2.5–10	125–250
	Mentalis	2.5–5	2.5–10	125–250
	Platysma	2.5–5	2.5–15	500–2500
	Zygomaticus	2.5–5	2.5–10	125–500
Jaw-closing dystonia	Masseter	40/site	20–60/site	1000–3000/site
	Temporalis	20/site	20–40/site	1000–3000/site
Jaw-opening dystonia	Pterygoids	5–20	5–20	1000–3000/site
	Digastric	5–15	5–15	250–750/site
Cervical dystonia				
• Anterocollis	Sternocleidomastoid	40	40–70	1000–3000
• Retrocollis	Splenius capitis	60	50–150	1000–5000
	Trapezius	60	50–150	1000–5000
• Torticollis (chin deviation)	Ipsilateral splenius capitis	60	50–150	1000–5000
	Contralateral sternocleidomastoid	40	40–70	1000–3000
• Laterocollis (head tilt)	Scalenes	30	15–50	1000–3000
• Shoulder elevation	Levator scapulae	80	25–100	1000–4000
	Trapezius	60	50–150	1000–5000
Shoulder abduction	Deltoid	50	50–150	

continued

TABLE 6.7 (cont.)

Presentation	Muscle	Average starting dose (Botox) (U)	Average dose (Botox) (U)	Starting Dose Range (Myobloc) (U)
Shoulder adduction	Pectoralis complex	100	75–150	2500–5000
	Latissimus dorsi	100	50–150	2500–5000
Elbow extension	Triceps	50	25–100	
Elbow flexion	Biceps	100	50–150	2500–5000
	Brachialis	60	40–100	1000–3000
	Brachioradialis	60	40–100	1000–3000
Wrist flexion	Flexor carpi radialis†	50	25–100	1000–3000
	Flexor carpi ulnaris†	40	20–70	1000–3000
Wrist extension	Extensor carpi radialis	20	25–100	500–1500
	Extensor carpi ulnaris†	20	20–40	500–1500
Wrist pronation	Pronator quadratus†	25	10–50	1000–2500
	Pronator teres†	40	25–75	1000–2500
Wrist supination	Supinator	20	15–45	
Finger flexion	Finger digitorum profundus†	20	20–40	1000–3000
	Finger digitorum superficialis†	20	20–40	1000–3000
Fisting	Flexor carpi radialis†	50	25–100	1000–3000
	Flexor carpi ulnaris†	40	20–70	1000–3000
	Extensor carpi ulnaris	20	10–30	500–1500
	Extensor carpi radialis	20	15–40	500–1500
	Finger digitorum profundus†	20	20–40	1000–3000
	Finger digitorum superficialis†	20	20–40	1000–3000

TABLE 6.7 (cont.)

Presentation	Muscle	Average starting dose (Botox) (U)	Average dose (Botox) (U)	Starting Dose Range (Myobloc) (U)
	Flexor pollicis longus†	20	10–30	1000–2500
	Opponens pollicis†	5	2.5–10	500–1500
Finger extension	Extensor indicis	5	2.5–10	500–1000
Thumb extension	Extensor pollicis longus	5	2.5–10	
Thumb-in-palm	Flexor pollicis longus†	20	10–30	1000–2500
	Opponens pollicis†	5	2.5–10	500–1500
	Adductor pollicis†			500–2500
Thumb protrusion	Extensor pollicis longus	5	2.5–10	
	Abductor pollicis longus	5	5–15	
Little finger abduction	Abductor digiti minimi	5	2.5–10	125–250
Flexed hip	Iliopsoas	150	50–200	3000–7500
	Rectus femoris	100	75–200	2500–5000
Hip adduction	Adductor magnus/longus/brevis	200	75–300	5000–10,000
Flexed knee	Semimembranosus	100	50–200	2500–7500
	Semitendinosus	100	50–200	2500–7500
	Biceps femoris	100	50–200	2500–7500
	Gastrocnemius	150	50–200	3,000–7500
Extended knee	Rectus femoris	100	75–200	3000–7500
	Vastus lateralis	100	50–200	3000–7500
	Vastus medialis	100	50–200	3000–7500
Plantar flexion (equinus)	Gastrocnemius	100	50–200	3000–7500
	Soleus	100	50–200	2500–5000
Foot inversion	Tibialis posterior	75	50–150	3000–7500
Foot dorsiflexion	Tibialis anterior	75	50–150	2500–5000

continued

TABLE 6.7 (cont.)

Presentation	Muscle	Average starting dose (Botox) (U)	Average dose (Botox) (U)	Starting Dose Range (Myobloc) (U)
Toe flexion	Flexor digitorum longus	75	50–100	2500–5000
	Flexor digitorum brevis	25	20–40	2500–5000
	Flexor hallucis longus	50	25–75	1500–3500
Striatal toe	Extensor hallucis longus	50	20–100	2000–4000

*Not considered a form of dystonia, even though it can cause blepharospasm and facial spasms; it is consistently unilateral. It is defined as a neurologic disorder manifested by involuntary, recurrent twitches of the eyelids, perinasal, perioral, zygomaticus, platysma, and other muscles of only one side of the face. It is usually due to a compression or irritation of the facial nerve by an aberrant artery or abnormal vasculatures around the brainstem. While microvascular decompression of the facial nerve has a high success rate, it also has risks such as permanent facial paralysis, stroke, and deafness, making botulinum toxin injection the treatment of choice.

†Start with lower doses if injecting these muscles for upper limb dystonia; doses provided are recommended for upper limb spasticity.

- Myobloc (comes in premixed 2500/5000/10,000 U vials).

- Maximum dose recommendations:

  - Recommended maximum dose per injection site is 50 U Botox.

  - Recommended maximum volume per site is 0.5 mL.

  - Should try not to reinject sooner than 3 months.

  - The adult recommended maximum dose/visit is 400 U of Botox.

  - In children:

    - The total maximum body dose/visit = the lesser of 12 U per kg or 400 U of Botox.

    - For large muscles, the recommended maximum should be no more than 3–6 U/kg of Botox.

- For small muscles, the recommended maximum should be no more than 1–2 U/kg of Botox.

■ Botulinum toxin dose modifiers (Table 6.8):

3. Surgical therapies:

■ Peripheral surgical procedures:

  ■ Rhizotomy

  ■ Ramisectomy

  ■ Myotomy

  ■ Intrathecal baclofen

■ CNS ablative procedures (see Chapter 9)

  ■ Pallidotomy

  ■ Thalamotomy

■ Deep brain stimulation (see also Chapter 9)

  ■ GPI stimulation

  ■ Ventrolateral thalamic stimulation

TABLE 6.8
Dose Modifiers to Consider When Injecting Botulinum Toxin

Clinical situation	Starting dose: low end of the range	Starting dose: high end of the range
Patient weight	Low	High
Patient age	Elderly	young
Muscle bulk	Very small	Very large
Number of regions injected	Many	Few
Disease severity/ dystonic spasms	Mild	Severe
Concern for weakness	High	Low
Results of previous therapy	Too much weakness	Inadequate denervation
Likely duration of therapy	Chronic	Acute

4. Other therapies:

■ Limb immobilization, focal splinting

■ Support groups

■ Physical therapy (gait, transfers, strengthening, stretching)

■ Occupational therapy (assistive devices to regain some independence)

REFERENCES

1. Fahn S. The varied clinical expressions of dystonia. Neurol Clin 1984;2:541–554.

2. Nutt JG, Muenter MD, Aronson A, et al. Epidemiology of focal and generalized dystonia in Rochester, Minnesota. Mov Disord 1988;3:188–194.

3. Marsden CD. The focal dystonias. Clin Neuropharmacol 1986;9:(Suppl 2):S49–60.

4. Fahn S. Generalized dystonia: concept and treatment. Clin Neurophramacol 1986; 9(Suppl 2):S37–S48.

5. Chan J, Brin MF, Fahn S. Idiopathic cervical dystonia: clinical characteristics. Mov Disord 1991;6:119–126.

6. Ozelius LJ, Hewett JW, Page CE, et al. The early onset torsion dystonia gene (DYT1) encodes at ATP binding protein. Nat Gene 1997;17:40–48.

7. Khan NL, Wood NW, Bhatia KP. Autosomal recessive DYT2-like primary torsion dystonia: a new family. Neurology 2003;61:1801–1803.

8. Nolte D, Niemann S, Muller U. Specific sequence changes in multiple transcript system DYT3 are associated with X-linked dystonia parkinsonism. Proc Natl Acad Sci USA 2003;100:10347–10352.

9. Parker N. Hereditary whispering dystonia. J Neurol Neurosurg Psychiatry 1985; 45:218–224.

10. Ichinose H, Ohye T, Takahashi E, et al. hereditary progressive dystonia with marked diurnal fluctuation caused by mutations in the GTP cyclohydrolase I gene. Nat Genet 1994;8: 236–242.

11. Almasy L, Bressman SB, Raymond D, et al. Idiopathic torsion dystonia linked to chromosome 8 in two Mennonite families. Ann Neurol 1997;42:670–673.

12. Leube B, Rudnicki D, Ratzlaff T, et al. Isiopathic torsion dystonia; assignment of a gene to chromosome 18p in a German family with adult onset, autosomal dominant inheritance and purely focal distribution. Hum Mol Genet 1996;5:1673–1677.

13. Fouad GT, Servidei S, Durcan S, et al. A gene for familial paroxysmal dyskinesia (FPD1) maps to chromosome 2q. Am J Hum Genet 1996;59:135–139.

14. Fink JK, Rainier S, Wilkowski J, et al. Paroxysmal dystonic choreoathetosis: tight linkage to chromosome 2q. Am J Hum Genet 1996;59:140–145.

15. Auburger G, Ratzlaff T, Lunkes A, et al. A gene for autosomal dominant paroxysmal choreoathetosis spasticity maps to the vicinity of a potassium channel gene cluster on chromosome 1p. Genomics 1996;31:90–94.

16. Tomita H, Nagamitsu S, Wakui K, et al. Paroxysmal kinesogenic choreoathetosis locus maps to chromosome 16p11.2-q12.1. Am J Hum Genet 1999;65:1688–1697.

17. Zimprich A, Grabowski M, Asmus F, et al. Mutations in the gene encoding epsilon-sarcoglycan cause myoclonus-dystonia syndrome. Nat Genet 2001; 29:66–69.

18. Kramer PL, Mineta M, Klein C, et al. Rapid onset dystonia parkinsonism: linkage to chromosome 19q13. Ann Neurol 1999;46:176–182.

19. Valente EM, Bentivoglio AR, Cassetta E, et al. DYT 13, a novel primary torsion dystonia locus maps to chromosome 1p36.13-36.32 in an Italian family with cranial-cervical or upper limb onset. Ann Neurol 2001;49:362–366.

20. Grotzsch H, Pizzolato GP, Ghika J, et al. Neuropathology of a case of dopa-responsive dystonia associated with new genetic locus, DYT 14. Neurology 2002; 58:1839–1842.

21. Grimes DA, Han F, Lang AE, et al. A novel locus for inherited myoclonus dystonia on 18p11. Neurology 2002;59:1183–1186.

22. Preston DC, Finkleman RS, Munsat TL, Dystonia postures generated from complex repetitive discharges. Neurology 1996;46:257–258.

7

THE "TIC" PATIENT

PHENOMENOLOGY

A tic is an involuntary movement or vocalization that is usually sudden onset, brief, repetitive, stereotyped but nonrhythmical in character, frequently imitating normal behavior, often occurring out of a background of normal activity. Tics are usually associated with a premonitory sensation or "build-up" sensation to perform the specific movement, and usually are associated with the sensation of relief once performed.

Tics can be classified as motor or vocal. Motor tics are associated with movements, while vocal tics are associated with sounds. Tics can also be categorized as *simple* or *complex*, depending on the manifestation (Table 7.1). Simple motor tics involve only a few muscles usually restricted to a specific body part. They can be clonic (abrupt in onset and rapid), tonic (isometric contraction of the involved body part), or dystonic (sustained abnormal posture).[1] Examples of simple motor tics include include:

- Eye blinking
- Shoulder shrugging
- Facial grimacing
- Neck stretching
- Mouth movements
- Jaw clenching

TABLE 7.1
Simple vs. Complex Tics

Type	Examples	Characteristics
Simple motor tics	Eye blinking, shoulder shrugging, facial grimacing, neck stretching, spitting, hair combing	Involve only one body region; only a few muscles used
Simple vocal tics	Throat clearing, grunting, coughing, sniffing	Sounds that do not form words
Complex motor tics	Jumping, kicking, squatting, abnormal body postures, echopraxia, copopraxia	Multiple body regions involved
Complex vocal tics	Coprolalia, palilalia, formed words, echolalia	Pronunciation of words or sentences, repetition of other people's words

■ Spitting

■ Hair combing

Simple vocal tics consist of sounds that do not form words, such as:

■ Throat clearing

■ Grunting

■ Coughing

■ Sniffing

Sometimes, the distinction between a motor and vocal tic may be difficult as the noise may result from a muscle contraction (see Table 7.1).

■ Complex motor tics

■ Consist of movements involving multiple muscle groups and have a deliberate character, frequently resembling normal movements or gestures.

■ Usually have a longer duration compared with simple tics.

■ Examples include jumping, kicking, squatting, or holding the body in atypical body positions.

■ May consist of imitating other people's gestures (echopraxia) or vulgar or obscene gesturing (copopraxia), such as exposing the person's genitalia.

- Complex vocal tics

  - Include pronunciation of words or sentences, repetition of other people words (echolalia), repetition of the last words or parts of the word (palilalia), or verbalizing profanities (coprolalia).

CHARACTERISTICS

- Tics are commonly associated with a premonitory sensation or discomfort that is usually relieved by performing the specific activity and typically will not disrupt volitional movement (differentiating tics from other abnormal movements such as chorea and myoclonus, which may share similarities with tics).

- Tics can be suppressed in many cases, but this usually will require concentration on the part of the affected individual and results in build-up of a "discomfort sensation" that is relieved by performance of the tic.

- The severity of tic performance usually waxes and wanes, with the individual experiencing episodes of repeated tic execution mixed with tic-free periods that may last from minutes to hours.[2]

- Involvement in activities that requires a great deal of attention or concentration usually diminishes the tic frequency, while worsening usually occurs in periods of stress or fatigue.

- Tics usually begin during childhood. The average onset of symptoms ranges from 5.6 years to 6.4 years and they become most severe at the age of 10 years, decreasing in frequency to the point that at 18 years, half of the patients suffering from tics are tic free.[3] The incidence of Tourette's syndrome (TS) is higher in males, with a male to female ratio of 4.3:1.[4] Rarely will the tics begin in adulthood, most frequently being recurrences of tics that occurred during childhood.[5]

- A common initial tic in TS patients is a facial tic. From here, movements may spread to involve the arms, trunk, and other body parts. Frequently, the tic is incorporated with other movements to make them look normal. In some patients, some tics may have a "violent" character that may result in increased morbidity.

The *Diagnostic and Statistical Manual of Mental Disorders,* 4th edition (DSM-IV), divides tic disorders in three main categories: transient tic disorders (TTDs), chronic motor or vocal tic disorder, and Tourette's disorder (Table 7.2).[6]

TABLE 7.2
DSM-IV Categories of Tic Disorders

Transient tic disorder	Single or multiple motor and/or vocal tics (i.e., sudden, rapid, recurrent, nonrhythmic, stereotyped motor movements or vocalizations) A. The tics occur many times a day, nearly every day for at least 4 weeks, but for no longer than 12 consecutive months. B. The onset is before age 18 years. C. The disturbance is not due to the direct physiologic effects of a substance (e.g., stimulants) or a general medical condition (e.g., Huntington's disease or postviral encephalitis). D. Criteria have never been met for Tourette's Disorder or Chronic Motor or Vocal Tic Disorder. Specify if single episode or recurrent	This is a diagnosis that is usually made in retrospect.
Chronic motor or vocal tic disorder	A. Single or multiple motor or vocal tics (i.e., sudden, rapid, recurrent, nonrhythmic, stereotyped motor movements or vocalizations), but not both, have been present at some time during the illness. B. The tics occur many times a day nearly every day or intermittently throughout a period of more than 1 year, and during this period there was never a tic-free period of more than 3 consecutive months. C. The onset is before age 18 years. D. The disturbance is not due to the direct physiologic effects of a substance (e.g., stimulants) or a general medical condition (e.g., Huntington's disease or postviral encephalitis). E. Criteria have never been met for Tourette's Disorder.	The tics in chronic tic disorders may wax and wane in severity and duration and during the course of the disease.
Tourette's syndrome	A. Both multiple motor and one or more vocal tics have been present at some time during the illness, although not necessarily concurrently. (A *tic* is a sudden, rapid, recurrent, nonrhythmic, stereotyped motor movement or vocalization.) B. The tics occur many times a day (usually in bouts) nearly every day or intermittently throughout a period of more than 1 year, and during this period there was never a tic-free period of more than 3 consecutive months. C. The onset is before age 18 years.	Abnormal activity must be witnessed by the examiner or evidence must be recorded by videotape.

TABLE 7.2 (cont.)

	D. The disturbance is not due to the direct physiologic effects of a substance (e.g., stimulants) or a general medical condition (e.g., Huntington's disease or postviral encephalitis).	
Tic disorder not otherwise specified	This category is for disorders characterized by tics that do not meet criteria for a specific Tic Disorder. Examples include tics lasting less than 4 weeks or tics with an onset after age 18 years.	

Associated Features

Two behavioral features commonly associated with TS are attention deficit–hyperactivity disorder (ADHD) and obsessive compulsive disorder (OCD). The incidence of ADHD in TS ranges between 50 and 75% and is the most common reported comorbidity. OCD may be seen in 30–60% of TS patients. For ADHD, the symptoms begin approximately 2.5 years before the onset of TD, while OCD is generally seen after tic onset.[8] Table 7.3 lists the symptoms seen with TS.

EPIDEMIOLOGY, PATHOGENESIS, AND PATHOPHYSIOLOGY

■ The prevalence of tic disorders shows dramatic variation, probably as a result of studied populations along with

TABLE 7.3
Other Symptoms Associated with TS

	Temper
Attention deficit and hyperactivity disorder	Short Temper
Obsessive-compulsive disorder	Oppositional defiant behavior
Confrontation	Mania
Violence	Agoraphobia
Anger	Simple phobia
Depression	Social phobia
Personality disorder	Problems with discipline

the diagnostic criteria and methodology used in different studies.

- For all tic disorders, the prevalence may be as high as 4.2%.[9] The prevalence of transient tic disorder has been reported to range from 4–24% and for TS 3%.[10]

- The exact origins of tics and TS are unknown, but it has been hypothesized that they involve the striatothalamocortical circuitry.

- Abnormalities in several neurotransmitter systems, particularly dopamine,[11] have been linked to the etiology of the syndrome.

- Despite contradictory findings seen in functional magnetic resonance imaging (MRI) studies, metabolic derangements have been detected in the orbitofrontal cortex, dorsolateral prefrontal cortex, supplementary motor areas, cingulate, sensorimotor cortex, and basal ganglia in other modalities, consistent with the idea that TS is both a motor and behavioral disorder.[12]

- Other reports link TS, ADHD, and OCD to previous infection with group A β-hemolytic streptococci, in what has been known as pediatric autoimmune neuropsychiatric disorders associated with streptococcus (PANDAS)[13] or other infectious agents.[14] The topic of PANDAS is highly controversial as many authors believe all of these cases to be TS.

- The occurrence of TS in family clusters suggest that TS has a genetic/familial basis. (Fifty-three percent pairwise concordance for TS in monozygotic twins, in contrast to 8% observed for dizygotic twins.)

- Multiple investigators have suggested an autosomal dominant with reduced penetrance mode of inheritance, and numerous candidate genes have been proposed, but to date there have been no significant linkage findings.

DIAGNOSTIC WORKUP

- The diagnoses of tics and TS are clinical ones. Table 7.4 lists the differential diagnosis for tics.

- There is no blood work or imaging studies that will confirm the diagnoses.

- Once the diagnoses are suspected, screening for behavioral symptoms should be performed and treatment should be initiated if necessary.

TABLE 7.4
Differential Diagnosis of Tics

Stereotype	Repetitive, purposeless movements	Rocking, shuddering, clapping, flapping, facial movements	Seen in normal children, also autism and developmental delays and pervasive developmental disorders
Compulsive behavior	Repetitive and ritualistic movements that usually are a response to psychologic need	Hand washing, repetitive cleaning, organizing in a particular manner	Seen in normal individuals or individuals with developmental delay. Obssesive thoughts may also be present
Punding	Stereotypical motor behavior in which there is an intense fascination with repetitive handling and examining of mechanical objects, such as picking at oneself or taking apart watches and radios or sorting and arranging of common objects, such as lining up pebbles, rocks, or other small objects[7]	Originally described in amphetamine users, now often reported in Parkinson's disease patients as a dopaminergic-induced complication	May be socially disruptive; responds to medication readjustment
Mannerism	Particular voluntary movement usually associated with a gesture or other particular movements	Example is rubbing hair after taking hat off, or extending the little finger when holding a cup. These movements may have a purpose	Nonpathologic actions that can often be a distinguishing feature of an individual
Seizure	Involuntary movement, may be associated with or without alteration of conciousness	Action varies depending of body region affected; EEG helpful for diagnosis	Nonsuppressible. Look for alteration in conciousness
Myoclonus	Sudden, brief, involuntary muscle jerk	May involve any body part, nonsuppressible	Myoclonus can resemble simple motor tics but are nonsuppressible and often random

continued

TABLE 7.4 (cont.)

Akathisia	Sensation of excessive restlessness resulting in constant movement of affected body parts, with relief upon moving	Leg movements, legs rubbing, walking, face rubbing. Affected individual cannot sit still	Associated with exposure to dopamine receptor–blocking agents (tardive akathisia), no diurnal fluctuation
Restless legs syndrome	Uncomfortable sensation, usually in lower extremities, happening in the afternoon or evening, relieved by movement	Patients describe symptoms differently: such as cramp, spasm, numbness, tingling, crawling sensation	The circadian nature suggests the diagnosis; improvement with dopamine agonist, levodopa, or narcotics

- If the patient is currently taking any medications, review them as some medications may be associated with induction of tics, including antidepressant medications and anticonvulsive agents.

- If a neurologic abnormality is found on examination, further workup should be undertaken to evaluate for secondary causes of tics (Table 7.5).

TREATMENT (Figure 7.1)

- Pharmacologic treatment for tics may not be needed unless they cause severe interference with school, work, or social development.

- Most patients with mild symptoms will benefit from education regarding the diagnosis and what to expect from the condition.

- Education should be extended to parents as well as teachers to create a suitable environment for the affected individual and explain to them that a tic disorder is not a mental disorder.

TABLE 7.5
Secondary Causes of Tics

Precipitants
Psychostimulants
Anticonvulsants
Anticholinergics
Antidepressants
CO intoxication
Head trauma
Genetic/chromosomal disorders
Huntington's disease
Neuroacanthocytosis
Encephalitis
Cardiopulmonary bypass

- Giving the affected child the opportunity to "release" the tics by providing her or him with a scheduled break may be all that is needed. The same may work for adults in the work environment.

- A behavioral treatment called habit reversal therapy has been reported as succesful in some centers, but this therapy remains under investigation.

If medical therapy is neccesary, the following should be considered:

- Therapy should be instituted taking into consideration the potential side effects.

- The focus of medical therapy relies on decreasing the impairment that is created by the tics rather than attempting to suppress them completely.

- The goal should be to begin therapy at low dosages and titrate to the lowest effective dosage.

- The mainstay of treatment for tics and TS are the dopamine receptor–blocking agents (Table 7.6).

  - Haloperidol and pimozide are probably the most widely used medications, and provide benefit to up to 80% of patients.

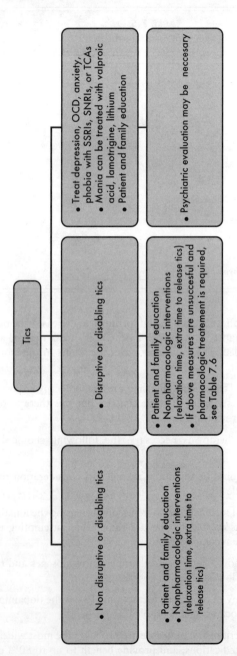

FIGURE 7.1

Approach to the management of the tic patient. Obsessive-compulsive disorder (OCD); selective serotonin reuptake inhibitors (SSRI); selective norepinephrine reuptake inhibitors (SNRI); and tricyclic antidepressants (TCA).

TABLE 7.6
Common Medications Used for the Treatment of Tics in TS

Generic Name	Dosing (mg/day)	Adverse Effects	Comments
Risperidone	0.25–6 qd-bid	TD, dizziness, sedation, akathisia, EPS	Begining with 0.25 mg at bedtime, increase every 3 days by 0.25 mg to benefit or side effects, risk of EPS > 6 mg/d
Haloperidol	0.5–5 mg bid-tid (adults) 0.05–0.075 mg/kg/d bid-tid (children)	Sedation, TD, EPS, NMS, galactorrhea, akathisia	Monitor for EPS
Olanzapine	2.5–20 mg qd	Weight gain, EPS, sedation, Diabetes mellitus, NMS, TD	Monitor for EPS and glucose
Pimozide	1–10 mg/d	ECG changes, weigth gain, EPS, sedation, TD	Check ECG at baseline, then periodically (prolongation of QT interval)
Quetiapine	25–800 mg/d	Weight gain, dizziness, drowsiness, hypotension, EPS	
Fluphenazine	1–10 mg/d	Sedation, TD, EPS, NMS, galactorrhea, akathisia	Better tolerated than haloperidol in some reports
Clonidine	0.05–0.6 mg/d, qd-bid	Sedation, hypotension, rebound hypertension with discontinuation, confusion	Start with low dose, monitor for hypotension, avoid abrupt withdrawal
Clonazepam or other benzodiazepines	Depending on the the benzodiazepine	Sedation, tolerance, cognitive impairment	Should not be used as first line; start with a low dose if possible

TD, *tardive dyskinesia;* EPS, *extrapyaramidal syndrome;* NMS, *neuroleptic malignant syndrome;* ECG, *electrocardiogram;* qd, *once daily;* bid, *twice daily*

- Fluphenazine has also been reported to be beneficial for tics, among others, in patients intolerant of haloperidol.

- Atypical antipsychotics have also been reported to be beneficial and may be associated with a lower incidence off side effects when compared with the typical antipsychotics.

  - Aripiprazole, risperidone, olazapine, quetiapine, amilsupride, ziprasidone, and sulpiride have been reported to decrease tic severity and frequency in multiple reports.

- Other treaments reported to be beneficial to reduce tic frequency in patients with TS include:

  - Nicotine

  - Mecamylamine, a nicotinic, acetylcholine anatagonist

  - Tetrabenazine

  - Tetrahydrocannabinol

  - Benzodiazepines, in particular clonazepam

  - Baclofen

  - Botulinum toxin

  - Clonidine and guanfacine

In recent years, reports of improvement with deep brain stimulation (DBS) in medically refractrory TS patients have been published, although there does not seem to be a consensus on the best target for electrode placement. Although still in the experimental phase, DBS may be a viable option for medically refractory patients with TS.

- Particular attention should be paid to the associated behavioral features, as they may become the most disabling aspect of the disease. Tretament for depression, anxiety, and obsessive-compulsive disorder with a selective serotonin reuptake inhibitor (SSRI) may be required and may be all that is needed. ADHD should be treated accordingly.

REFERENCES

1. Jankovic J. Tourette syndrome. Phenomenology and classification of tics. Neurol Clin 1997;15(2):267–275.
2. Peterson BS, Leckman JF. The temporal dynamics of tics in Gilles de la Tourette syndrome. Biol Psychiatry 1998;44(12):1337–1348.
3. Diagnostic and Statistical Manual of Mental Disorders (DSM-IV-TR). Washington DC: American Psychiatric Association, 2000.

4. Leckman JF, Zhang H, Vitale A, et al. Course of tic severity in Tourette syndrome: the first two decades. Pediatrics 1998;102(1 Pt 1): 14–19.

5. Freeman RD, Fast DK, Burd L, et al. An international perspective on Tourette syndrome: selected findings from 3,500 individuals in 22 countries. Dev Med Child Neurol 2000;42(7):436–447.

6. Chouinard S, Ford B. Adult onset tic disorders. J Neurol Neurosurg Psychiatry 2000;68(6):738–43.

7. Fernandez HH, Friedman JH. Punding on L-dopa. Mov Disord 1999;14(5):836–838.

8. Shapiro AK SE, Young JG, et al. Gilles de la Tourette Syndrome, 2nd ed. New York: Raven Press, 1988.

9. Costello EJ, Angold A, Burns BJ, et al. The Great Smoky Mountains Study of Youth. Goals, design, methods, and the prevalence of DSM-III-R disorders. Arch Gen Psychiatry 1996;53(12):1129–1136.

10. Mason A, Banerjee S, Eapen V, et al. The prevalence of Tourette syndrome in a mainstream school population. Dev Med Child Neurol 1998;40(5):292–296.

11. Kurlan R. Tourette's syndrome: current concepts. Neurology 1989;39(12):1625–1630.

12. Adams JR, Troiano AR, Calne DB. Functional imaging in Tourette's syndrome. J Neural Transm 2004;111(10–11):1495–1506.

13. Muller N, Kroll B, Schwarz MJ, et al. Increased titers of antibodies against streptococcal M12 and M19 proteins in patients with Tourette's syndrome. Psychiatry Res 2001;101(2):187–193.

14. Muller N, Riedel M, Blendinger C, et al. Mycoplasma pneumoniae infection and Tourette's syndrome. Psychiatry Res 2004;129(2): 119–125.

8

THE "UNSTEADY" PATIENT

ROLE OF THE CEREBELLUM

The cerebellum modulates functions that are generated in other areas of the brain. As a motor modulator, the cerebellum has two functions:

1. It balances contractile forces of muscles during motor activity.

2. It organizes complex motor actions.

Different regions of the cerebellum have different functions. Table 8.1 delineates the function of various cerebellar divisions.

Table 8.1
Cerebellar Functional Divisions

Phylogenetic origin	Anatomic location	Function modulated
Archicerebellum	*Midline* Flocculonodular lobe	Vestibular function Eye movements
Paleocerebellum	*Midline* Vermis (anterior lobe) Pyramis Uvula Paraflocculus	Muscle tone Axial control Stance Gait
Neocerebellum	*Midline/hemispheres* Middle vermis Cerebellar hemispheres	Movement initiation, planning Fine motor programs Possibly cognition

ANATOMIC/FUNCTIONAL CORRELATIONS

A few brief key anatomic facts are useful in understanding the clinical findings of cerebellar dysfunction (Table 8.2).

CLINICAL MANIFESTATIONS OF CEREBELLAR DYSFUNCTION

Cerebellar dysfunction parallels cerebellar phylogenetic organization.

- Midline cerebellar dysfunction involves axial control, including vestibular function, eye movements, balance, and postural stability.

- Hemispheric cerebellar deficits impact motor planning and control of fine motor movements.

Table 8.2
Key Functional and Anatomic Facts

Remember	Because	Implications
Location	The cerebellum is located in close proximity to vital brain structures.	A swelling cerebellum or cerebellar mass can cause hydrocephalus. A swelling cerebellum or cerebellar mass can displace other brain structures, causing herniation.
Anatomy	The hemispheres coordinate the arms and legs. The midline coordinates the trunk (balance).	Lesions in the hemispheres result in limb ataxia. Lesions in the midline result in gait and balance problems, truncal titubation, and wide-based gait.
Decussation	The cerebellum features a double decussation.	Lesions of the left cerebellum affect the left side. Lesions of the right cerebellum affect the right side.
Function	The cerebellum is a motor modulator.	Ataxia and gait problems can result not just from lesions of the cerebellum, but also lesions of the input and output pathways. 1. Spinal sensory afferents (routed mainly through the medulla) 2. Cortical motor afferents (routed through the pons) 3. Thalamic output pathways (routed through the midbrain)

- Data regarding the impact of cerebellar modulation on general cognitive function is still emerging, but the cerebellum may have an impact on planning, organizing, and sequencing executive planning functions that parallels its impact on motor planning and fine motor programs.[1]

- Table 8.3 outlines simple bedside clinical examination techniques in patients with suspected cerebellar dysfunction. Depending on the severity of the deficit and localization of the lesion, some deficits will be evident on examination, while others may be subtle or not present.

CLASSIFICATION AND DIAGNOSTIC WORKUP

Diagnosis of ataxic syndromes is becoming increasingly challenging. A complete history, physical examination, neuroimaging, as well as extensive laboratory evaluation are required. In many cases, the etiology of ataxia remains uncertain despite a complete workup.

- Many chronic cerebellar ataxias are genetically determined, and family history should be obtained. Many genetic ataxic syndromes can feature "anticipation," a progressively lower age of onset in successive generations (family history may be absent in some individuals). In some cases, presentation of a similar syndrome in a sibling despite unaffected parents may be an important clue. Patients should be asked about consanguinity (e.g., are your parents related in any way?), as this can sometimes point to the possibility of recessively inherited disorders such as Friedreich's ataxia.

- Ataxia may also occur sporadically in disorders such as multiple system atrophy (MSA), a syndrome that can also present with autonomic instability and parkinsonism. In younger patients, nutritional abnormalities (some genetically related) such as primary vitamin E deficiency, as well as abnormalities in serum lipoproteins causing fat malabsorption can cause ataxia, as can mitochondrial disease. In older patients, autoimmune syndromes including paraneoplastic syndromes can result in ataxia. Celiac disease, an autoimmune disease with antigliadin antibodies, may result in ataxia.[2] Furthermore, ataxia can be associated with multiple sclerosis both as an acute or a chronic feature of the disease.

- With the proliferation of potential diagnoses with ataxia, clinicians should develop a careful and standardized approach

Table 8.3
Clinical Examination of the Ataxic Patient

Clinical domain	Examination technique	Finding with cerebellar dysfunction
Eye movements	Observation.	Macular square wave jerks (sudden, spontaneous, unplanned deviations of the eye with corrective saccades back to original position).
	Have the patient fixate on an object off midline (e.g., examiner's finger). Command: "Look at my finger here on the right . . . now on the left."	Fixation instability: Involuntary saccades away from object. Corrective saccades back to object. Nystagmus (fixation in lateral or vertical gaze): Fixation interrupted by slow rolling movements, often toward a neutral position, interrupted by rapid corrective saccades.
	Saccade between two objects (e.g., examiner's finger and nose). Command: "Look at my finger . . . now look at my nose . . . finger . . . nose."	Dysmetric saccades: Saccade may overshoot or undershoot the target, with a correction.
	Smooth pursuit of an object through space. Command: "Follow my finger through space."	The eyes should move smoothly. Saccadic fragmentation of smooth pursuit is a common finding in healthy elderly, but can also be a sign of cerebellar disease.
	Caveats	Vestibular dysfunction may cause nystagmus. Slight lateral nystagmus is common in healthy adults. Saccadic pursuit may occur in healthy elderly. Slowed saccades, inability to generate saccades, and opthalmoplegia may occur, but generally indicate additional brainstem involvement.
Tremor	Finger to nose testing and finger chasing, holding hands in horizontal posture.	Usually low frequency, but high-amplitude intention and postural tremor.

Table 8.3 (cont.)

Clinical domain	Examination technique	Finding with cerebellar dysfunction
Limb coordination	Finger to nose testing. Finger chasing (the examiner moves the finger and has the patient try to keep his or her finger behind the examiner's finger (mirroring).	Past pointing (missing examiner's finger). Excessive corrections. Rebound.
	Tapping heel to knee. Running heel from knee to shin.	Abnormal speed. Poor precision. Excessive corrections.
	Rapid alternating tapping (rapidly tapping palmar and dorsal aspect of hand on thigh).	Slowed movements with impaired precision. "Painting the leg" rather than tapping the leg.
Stance/gait	Observation of casual gait.	Unsteady, wide-based gait. Difficulty with sudden stops or changes in direction. Variable step length. Often patients will visually focus on the ground.
	Tandem gait.	More pronounced deficits, "steps to the side" to catch balance.
	Stance with eyes closed.	"Positive Romberg" = Abnormal sensory input or reception in the cerebellum. Patients are unable to maintain balance with eyes closed.
Muscle tone	Evaluate tone at wrist, elbow, knee, and ankle.	Deceased resistance to passive movement.
Speech evaluation	Prepared text may be helpful; e.g., "The Rainbow Passage"—See Appendix.	Altered articulation of words. Abnormal fluency. Slowed speech. "Scanning dysarthria"— words are broken into syllables.

to diagnosis (Figures 8.1 and 8.2). The time course of the ataxia is an important diagnostic feature, as acute ataxic syndromes frequently are related to acute infectious and vascular, structural, or metabolic lesions, while chronic ataxias are more apt to be related to genetic syndromes or slow-growing mass lesions. Possible algorithms for evaluation of ataxic syndromes in children and adults are presented in

Ataxia
Unsteadiness

Acute

Infectious
  Cerebellar abcess
  Brainstem viral encephalitis
  Viral labyrinthitis
  Acute cerebellitis (Varicella)
Benign positional vertigo
Head trauma or child abuse
  Posterior fossa hematoma
Metabolic or genetic
  Acute intoxication
  Mitochondrial
  Pyruvate decarboxylase
    deficiency
  Carnitine acyltransferase
    deficiency
  Hartnup disease
  Juvenile maple syrup urine
    disease
  Ornithine transcarbamoy-
    lase deficiency
  Familial episodic ataxia
Autoimmune, incl.
paraneoplastic
  Miller-Fischer variant of
    Guillain-Barré syndrome
  Acute demyelinating
    encephalomyopathy
    (ADEM)
  Multiple sclerosis
  Neuroblastoma
    (Opsoclonus-Myoclonus)
Vascular
  Ischemic stroke
  Intercerebral hemmorrhage
  Deep venous thrombosis
  Subarachnoid hemorrhage
Neoplasm
  Medulloblastoma
  Astrocytoma
  Ependymoma
  Metastasis

Diagnostic Workup

Complete neurologic
  examination
Complete physical exam, pulm
  function
Family/social history
CNS imaging (Head CT
  followed by MRI).
  May require arterial/venuous
  imaging
Consider: Lumbar puncture,
  toxin screen, lactate,
  pyruvate, serum and urine
  amino acids, serum organic
  acids, ammonia level

Episodic

Child abuse
  Acute head trauma
  Posterior fossa hematoma
Benign positional vertigo
Metabolic
  Drug ingestion
  Mitochondrial
  Pyruvate decarboxylase
    deficiency
  Carnitine acyltransferase
    deficiency
  Hartnup disease
  Juvenile maple syrup urine
    disease
  Ornithine transcarbamoylase
    deficiency
Neoplasm
  Medulloblastoma
  Astrocytoma
  Ependymoma
Genetic
  Familial episodic ataxia

Diagnostic Workup

Complete neurologic
  examination
Opthalmologic examination
Complete physical exam
Family/social history
CNS imaging (MRI).
  May require arterial/venous
  imaging
Consider: Lumbar puncture,
  toxin screen, lactate,
  pyruvate, serum and
  urine amino acids,
  serum organic acids,
  ammonia level, genetic testing
  (Episodic ataxia)

Chronic

Head trauma or abuse
Neoplasm
  Medulloblastoma
  Astrocytoma
  Ependymoma
Ataxic cerebral palsy
Structural
  Cerebellar hypoplasia
  Basilar impression
  Arnold chiari malformation
Multiple sclerosis
Metabolic or genetic
  Chronic substance abuse
  Vitamin E deficiency
  Leukodystrophy
  Childhood ataxia with CNS
    Hypomeylination (CACH)
  Autosomal dominant
    Spinocerebellar ataxia
  Autosomal recessive
    Abetalipoproteinemia
      (Vit E)
    Ataxia telangiectasia
    Friedreich's ataxia
    Juvenile GM2
      gangliosidosis
    Juvenile sulfatide lipidosis
    Marinesco-Sjorgen
      syndrome
    Juvenile nieman pick
      disease
    Refsum disease
Mitochondrial

Diagnositic Workup

Complete neurologic
  examination
Opthalmologic examination
Complete physical exam
Family/social history
CNS imaging (MRI).
  May require arterial/venous
  imaging
Serum toxin screen
Consider metabolic/genetic
  testing: Genetic testing for
  autosomal dominant ataxias
  and Friedreich's ataxia,
  Vitamin E, Vitamin B-12,
  serum lipoproteins, serum
  phytanic acid, serum alpha-
  fetoprotein, serum acid
  sphingomyelinase,
  hexosaminidase, urine
  sulfatide. Consider acute
  ataxia screening panel, as
  some acute causes of ataxia
  can result in chronic ataxia.

FIGURE 8.1
Diagnostic algorithm for the ataxic child/adolescent.

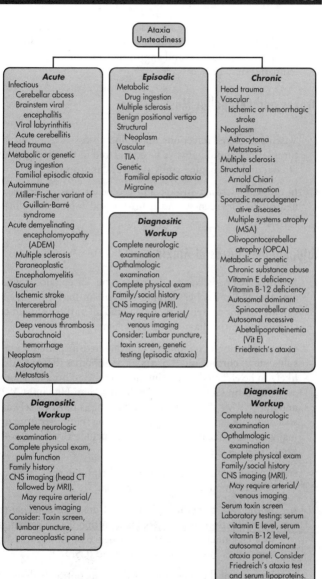

FIGURE 8.2
Diagnostic algorithm for the ataxic adult.

Figures 8.1 and 8.2. In some cases, certain genetic syndromes may be more common in a local population or family history may provide guidance, and appropriate modification of these templates may be necessary.

Strokes and Cerebellar Mass Lesions

■ Vascular lesions, infections (including abscesses), and structural lesions should always be considered in the diagnosis of ataxia, and an imaging study is always appropriate.

■ In an acute setting, strokes and cerebellar masses can be a neurologic emergency, and neurosurgical intervention may be required.

Autoimmune Causes of Ataxia

■ Multiple sclerosis, acute demyelinating encephalomyelitis, and the Miller-Fischer variant of Guillian-Barré syndrome can all present acutely with ataxia, and all of these should be considered in the diagnosis of acute ataxia.

■ Paraneoplastic ataxia should be evaluated in patients with subacute to chronic onset of ataxia. Antibodies that are most likely to be elevated in autoimmune cerebellar ataxia include anti-GQ1b (in Guillian-Barré syndrome),[3] anti-Hu, anti-CV-2, and anti-CRMP-5.[4] Paraneoplastic ataxia is most closely associated with small cell cancer of the lung, but other primary malignancies that may be associated include thymoma and, rarely, uterine sarcoma.

   ■ A lumbar puncture is frequently helpful in the diagnosis of autoimmune etiologies of ataxia.

   ■ In the case of paraneoplastic syndromes, in addition to an evaluation of paraneoplastic antibodies in serum, a lumbar puncture may reveal evidence of paraneoplastic antibodies in the cerebrospinal fluid (CSF).

   ■ Imaging of the chest and neck with a contrast-enhanced computed tomogram (CT) is indicated if there is a suspicion of a paraneoplastic syndrome.

Genetic Causes of Ataxia

In no area has the diagnosis of ataxia become more complex than in genetic causes of ataxia.

- Identifiable recessive causes of ataxia are more common in children, including a host of metabolic abnormalities such as juvenile forms of GM2 gangliosidoses, sulfatide lipidoses, and other syndromes involving deposition of abnormal metabolic intermediates.[5]

- Friedreich's ataxia can occur in children and in young adults, and has occasionally been described in older individuals.

- Hereditary ataxia with vitamin E deficiency is recessive and can present with symptoms very similar to those found in Friedreich's ataxia.[6,7]

- Abetalipoproteinemia is another recessive cause of vitamin E deficiency, and depending on the severity of the deficit and the related vitamin E deficiency, may occur in children or adults.[7]

- Case reports in the literature suggest that vitamin B_{12} may also occasionally present with chronic ataxia, often related to loss of proprioception.[8-9]

  - Vitamin E and vitamin B_{12} levels should be checked in all individuals with new onset of ataxia, as this is a potentially correctable cause of progressive ataxia.

- Table 8.4 lists some of the more frequently seen causes of recessive cerebellar ataxia, as well as clinical findings.

Episodic ataxia is a rare and defined dominantly inherited genetic entity. Two distinct presentations have been identified, and genetic tests are available.

1. In episodic ataxia 1 (EA1), episodes of ataxia, with gait imbalance and slurring of speech, occur spontaneously or can be precipitated by sudden movement, excitement, or exercise. The attacks generally last from seconds to several minutes at a time and may recur many times a day.

2. In episodic ataxia 2 (EA2), ataxia lasts hours to days, with interictal eye movement abnormalities. Exertion and stress commonly precipitate the episodes. EA2 notably is due to a genetic defect in a calcium channel (CACNA1A), and different genetic defects of this channel can cause genetically transmitted familial hemiplegic migraine.[7,10]

- A CAG repeat in this gene causes a progressive ataxia (SCA6), and there are overlaps in symptomatology.[11,12]

- Patients may have migrainous episodes as well as ataxia, and some patients with the SCA6 mutation may present with episodic ataxia.

Table 8.4
Autosomal Recessive Cerebellar Ataxias

Name	Gene product identified?	Available test?	Clinical findings
Friedreich's ataxia	Yes	Yes	Classically, juvenile ataxia with a proprioceptive neuropathy, but a wide variety of presentations have been described.
Hereditary ataxia with vitamin E deficiency	Yes	Yes	Ataxia with proprioceptive neuropathy, low vitamin E level.
Abetalipoproteinemia	Yes	Yes	Ataxia with proprioceptive neuropathy, low vitamin E level, abnormal serum lipoproteins.
X-linked ataxia with sideroblastic anemia	Yes	No	Slowly progressive childhood onset ataxia with sideroblastic anemia.
Ataxia-telangiectasia	Yes	Yes	Ataxia, chorea, dystonia, oculomotor apraxia.

- Acetazolamide may be helpful in the treatment of episodic ataxia.

  Potential identifiable causes of ataxia in individuals in whom there is a history suggestive of a dominant pedigree have proliferated.

- There are currently 24 identified causes of autosomal dominant ataxia, including seven syndromes caused by CAG repeats encoding a polyglutamine protein domain (SCA1, SCA2, SCA3, SCA6, SCA7, SCA17, DRPLA). Another five syndromes have other identified genetic causes.[13] Ongoing searches for the genetic locus and gene product in the other 12 syndromes are still ongoing. Currently, genetic testing is available for several of these disorders through a variety of sources.

  - Worldwide, approximately 65% of identified families with autosomal dominant ataxia have SCA1, SCA2, SCA3, SCA6, SCA7, or SCA8. Frequency of individual ataxic syndromes varies from one country to another.[14-15]

- Worldwide, SCA3 is the most common cause of autosomal dominant cerebellar ataxia, accounting for roughly 21% of identified families (see also Chapter 6).[13] SCA3 is even more common in Brazil, Germany, and China.

- SCA1 is more prevalent in Italy and South Africa.

- Dentatorubropallidoluysian atrophy (DRPLA), a disease with protean manifestations that can present with ataxia, is an uncommon cause of ataxia worldwide. The disease, however, is more prevalent in Japan (see also Chapters 2, 3, and 6)

- Although the state of the science is changing rapidly, currently ataxia with autosomal dominant inheritance has an unknown genetic cause in approximately 30% of affected families.[13]

In patients with onset of ataxia and with a family history, autosomal dominant ataxia should be considered. Table 8.5 identifies the major known autosomal dominant disorders and their genetic causes. A full discussion of the causes of autosomal dominant ataxias is beyond the scope of this chapter; however a few important points are relevant:

- Some causes of autosomal dominant ataxia result in a pure ataxic syndrome, while with others, spasticity, neuropathy, cognitive changes, dystonia, or parkinsonism may be an added feature. Identification of features outside of pure motor ataxia may be helpful in making a diagnosis of a specific disorder.

- Pursuing genetic testing of unaffected family members of individuals with a proven autosomal dominant spinocerebellar ataxia is a complex issue, and in many cases, a genetic counselor should be involved prior to testing.

- Autosomal dominant ataxias due to trinucleotide repeats, such as CAG repeats, have the characteristic of anticipation. Later generations may have expansion of the repeat and earlier onset of the disease. Offspring of male carriers are more likely to have a repeat expansion than offspring of female carriers.

- A special note is necessary with respect to SCA8. Although most cases of SCA8 appear to be associated with a CTG expansion, CTG expansions in the same region have been shown to occur in some healthy controls. Genetic testing should therefore be interpreted in this disorder with particular caution.

Table 8.5
Autosomal Dominant Cerebellar Ataxias

Name	Product identified?	Available test?	Clinical findings
SCA1	Yes	Yes	Ataxia, spasticity, executive dysfunction
SCA2	Yes	Yes	Ataxia, hyporeflexia, dementia, rare parkinsonism
SCA3	Yes	Yes	Ataxia, spasticity, dystonia, parkinsonism, restless legs, dementia
SCA4			Ataxia, spasticity, axonal sensory neuropathy
SCA5	Yes	Yes	Typically early onset ataxia with normal life expectancy
SCA6	Yes	Yes	Ataxia
SCA7	Yes	Yes	Ataxia, pigmentary retinopathy, spasticity
SCA8	Yes	Yes	Ataxia
SCA10	Yes	Yes	Ataxia, epilepsy
SCA11			Ataxia, normal life expectancy, occasional spasticity
SCA12	Yes	No	Ataxia, spasticity
SCA13			Often early onset (childhood) ataxia (but may occur later) with slow progression and normal life expectancy. Mental retardation
SCA14	Yes	Yes	Slowly progressive ataxia with normal life expectancy. Myoclonus if childhood onset
SCA15			Ataxia, occasional spasticity
SCA16			Ataxia, normal life expectancy, head tremor
SCA17	Yes	Yes	Ataxia, parkinsonism, dystonia, chorea, psychosis
SCA18			Ataxia, axonal neuropathy
SCA19			Ataxia, dementia, hyporeflexia or hyperreflexia
SCA21			Ataxia, dementia
SCA25			Ataxia, sensory neuropathy
FGF14	Yes	No	Ataxia, psychiatric abnormalities
DRPLA	Yes	Yes	Ataxia, myoclonus, epilepsy, chorea, psychosis, dementia

Sporadic Causes of Ataxia

Unexplained chronic progressive ataxia in adult patients without a family history is less likely to be genetic (however it is still possible).[16] One prominent cause of progressive ataxia in older adults is multiple system atrophy. Multiple system atrophy is a disease of unknown cause that can present with parkinsonism, postural hypotension, or primary ataxia. In many cases, patients may present with one finding and develop other neurologic manifestations over time. Dementia often develops late in the disorder. Pathophysiologically, the disease is characterized by loss of oligodendroglia and neurons in multiple structures throughout the brain. Progression is relatively rapid compared to many genetic causes of ataxia.

In patients with a chronic adult-onset ataxia, a cause for the ataxia may not be found. In a recent German study of 112 patients with chronic progressive ataxia (inclusion criteria included onset over age 20, progressive course, no identified symptomatic cause including no evidence of a paraneoplastic process, and no evidence of a family history of ataxia),[16] 58% were undiagnosed after an extensive workup. In 29%, patients met criteria for multiple system atrophy. Genetic testing revealed an autosomal dominant or recessive ataxia in 13% (SCA1, SCA2, SCA6, or adult-onset Friedreich's ataxia were identified during genetic screening in these individuals). In the 58% of patients for whom a diagnosis was not made, ataxia tended to have a slower rate of progression than multiple system atrophy.

TREATMENT

Acute cerebellar ataxia should be considered a neurologic emergency until certain diagnoses are excluded. Key facts to consider in the management of acute ataxia:

1. In children, metabolic abnormalities can be caused by inborn errors of metabolism, and rapid treatment may be required to prevent permanent brain injury.

2. Acute intoxications in children and adults can be fatal if not treated.

3. Vascular and structural cerebellar lesions such as strokes, hemorrhages, and neoplasms can result in swelling causing herniation or obstruction of CSF flow causing hydrocephalus, and neurosurgical interventions may be required.

4. The Miller-Fischer variant of Guillain-Barré syndrome can present with ataxia and dysarthria and cause deficits in upper airway function that can impair respiration.

5. In children, abuse should always be considered as a potential etiology for trauma.

In chronic ataxias, a complete family history should be performed. An autosomal dominant pattern of inheritance may be helpful in narrowing the differential diagnosis. There is currently no universal treatment for ataxia.

■ In some cases (paraneoplastic ataxia or ataxia due to an autoimmune disease, structural abnormality, nutritional deficiency, or metabolic abnormality), identification of the underlying cause of ataxia may also identify a treatment modality.

■ In many cases, treatment is supportive and includes physical therapy, occupational therapy, and speech therapy for patients impacted with dysarthria and dysphagia. A baseline speech and swallowing evaluation by a speech pathologist should be performed in most cases in all but the most mildly affected patients, even if there is not an overt swallowing deficit.

■ In the case of the genetically linked ataxias, genetic counseling is an important part of management, and testing of unaffected family members should be performed only with much care after providing full information to family members.

■ Several agents have been inconsistently reported to improve ataxia: amantadine, L-5-hydroxytryptophan, odansetron, physostigmine, branched-chain amino acid therapy, gabapentin, piracetam.

■ Surgical ablation or deep brain stimulation surgery of the ventral intermediate nucleus (VIN) of the thalamus may be effective in reducing cerebellar tremor; however, they often do not significantly lessen ataxia, although a few cases have been reported with benefit (e.g., SCAs).

Ataxia is a complex entity that can be the presenting feature of many different neurologic disorders. Evaluation and management of ataxia should focus first on excluding symptomatic causes. Consideration of genetic testing should occur after reversible causes are excluded. Acute onset of ataxia should be considered a neurologic and potentially a neurosurgical emergency until structural, vascular, or toxic causes of acute ataxia are ruled out. In children, reversible causes include a host of metabolic lesions that should be considered, and referral to a pediatric neurologist may be appropriate if initial evaluations are not fruitful. In adults, vitamin E and occasionally vitamin B_{12} deficiency are rarely a cause of chronic progressive ataxia and should not be overlooked in a diagnostic workup. After a careful symptomatic workup, consideration for testing for genetic causes of ataxia should be considered. In patients with an identified genetic cause, testing of unaffected family members should be performed with caution and the involvement of a genetic counselor is often helpful. After correction of symptomatic causes, management is typically supportive but may include physical, occupational, and speech therapy.

REFERENCES

1. Schmahmann JD, Caplan D. Cognition, emotion and the cerebellum. Brain. 2006;129(Pt 2):290–292.
2. Abele M, Schˆls L, Schwartz S, Klockgether T. Prevalence of antigliadin antibodies in ataxia patients. Neurology 2003;60:1674–1675.
3. Paparounas K. Anti-GQ1b ganglioside antibody in peripheral nervous system disorders. Pathophysiologic role and clinical relevance. Arch Neurol 2004;61:1013-1016.
4. Bataller L, Dalmau J. Paraneoplastic neurologic syndromes. Neurol Clin North Am 2003;21:221–247.
5. Berman P. Ataxia in children. Int Pediatr 1999;14(1):44-47.
6. Stocker A. Molecular mechanisms of vitamin E transport. Ann N Y Acad Sci 2004;1031:44–59.
7. van de Warrenburg BPC, Sinke RJ, Kremer B. Recent advances in hereditary spinocerebellar ataxias. J Neuropathol Exp Neurol 2005;64 (3):171–180.
8. Miller MA, Martinez V, McCarthy R, Patel MM. Nitrous oxide "whippit" abuse presenting as clinical B12 deficiency and ataxia. Am J Emerg Med 2004;22(2):124.
9. Morita S, Miwa H, Kihira T, Kondo T. Cerebellar ataxia and leukoencephalopathy associated with cobalamin deficiency. J Neurol Sci 2003;216(1):183–184.
10. Facchini SA, Jami MM, Neuberg RW, Sorrel AD. A treatable cause of ataxia in children. Pediatr Neurol 2001;24(2):135–138.
11. Ophoff RA, Terwindt GM, Vergouwe MN, et al. Familial hemiplegic migraine and episodic ataxia type-2 are caused by mutations in the Ca2+ channel gene CACNL1A4. Cell 1996;87:543–552.
12. Frontali M. Spinocerebellar ataxia type 6: channelopathy or glutamine repeat disorder? Brain Res Bull 2001;56:227–231.
13. Abele M, Burk K, Schols L, et al. The aetiology of sporadic adult-onset ataxia. Brain 2002;125(Pt 5):961–968.
14. Schöls L, Bauer P, Schmidt T, et al. Autosomal dominant cerebellar ataxias: clinical features, genetics, and pathogenesis. Lancet Neurol 2004;3:291–304.

15. van de Warrenburg BP, Sinke RJ, Verschuuren-Bemelmans CC, et al. Spinocerebellar ataxias in the Netherlands: prevalence and age at onset variance analysis. Neurology 2002;58:702–708.

16. Silveira I, Miranda C, Guimaraes L, et al. Trinucleotide repeats in 202 families with ataxia: a small expanded (CAG) nallele at the SCA17 locus. Arch Neurol 2002;59:623–629.

17. Brusco A, Gellera C, Cagnoli C, et al. Molecular genetics of hereditary spinocerebellar ataxia: mutation analysis of spinocerebellar ataxia genes and CAG/CTG repeat expansion detection in 225 Italian families. Arch Neurol 2004;61(5):727–733.

18. Bryer A, Krause A, Bill P, et al. The hereditary adult onset ataxias in South Africa. J Neurol Sci 2003;216:47–54.

19. Tang B, Liu C, Shen L, et al. Frequency of SCA1, SCA2, SCA3/MJD, SCA6, SCA7, and DRPLA CAG trinucleotide repeat expansion in patients with hereditary spinocerebellar ataxia from Chinese kindreds. Arch Neurol 2000 57:540–544.

20. Saleem Q, Choudhry S, Mukerji M, et al. Molecular analysis of autosomal dominant hereditary ataxias in the Indian population: high frequency of SCA2 and evidence for a common founder mutation. Hum Genet 2000;106:179–87.

21. Moseley ML, Benzow KA, Schut LJ, et al. Incidence of dominant spinocerebellar and Friedreich triple repeats among 361 ataxia families. Neurology 1998;51:1666–1671.

22. Abele M, Burk K, Schols L, et al. The aetiology of sporadic adult-onset ataxia. Brain 2002;125(Pt 5):961–968.

9

KEY CONCEPTS FOR SURGICAL THERAPY FOR PARKINSON'S DISEASE AND MOVEMENT DISORDERS

Deep brain stimulation (DBS) is a promising technology that has provided symptomatic relief for PD, dystonia, tremor, tics, and various other movement disorders. However, only a small number of patients referred to surgical centers may be excellent candidates for DBS. Recent Food and Drug Administration (FDA) approval of DBS for Parkinson's disease (PD), essential tremor, and dystonia has made these procedures widely available in the United States, but they are also available worldwide. The procedure, including screening, implantation, and follow-up, requires advanced training, specialty expertise, and a commitment of an interdisciplinary team to the care of implanted patients. Patients interested in DBS can receive the therapy from over 200 centers in North America, and many others around the world (but only a few offer surgery for dystonia because of FDA and institutional review board (IRB) restrictions. The content of this chapter aims to provide a useful framework for patients, general neurologists, and practitioners to screen and treat appropriate DBS candidates.

DBS can be performed unilaterally or bilaterally to treat medication-refractory PD symptoms (Figures 9.1 and 9.2).

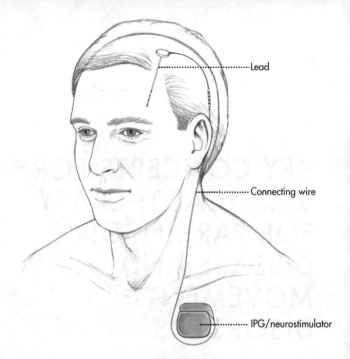

FIGURE 9.1
Unilateral DBG.

What Is Deep Brain Stimulation?

- DBS is a procedure that utilizes a lead that is implanted into "deep" brain structures. It may be used in place of or in conjunction with lesioning procedures such as pallidotomy or thalamotomy (burning a hole in structures in the brain that control movement).[1]

- Patients with PD, tremor, dystonia, or obsessive-compulsive disorder/Tourette's syndrome (OCD/Tourette) who are medically refractory to standard therapies, and who have no cognitive difficulties or "minimal" cognitive dysfunction, and who are otherwise healthy may qualify.

- The currently used lead is FDA approved and manufactured by the Medtronic Corporation, Minneapolis, Minnesota.

  - It has four electrode contacts (quadrapolar), and depending on the disorder and/or the target, one may use various sized contacts with different spacing arrangements.

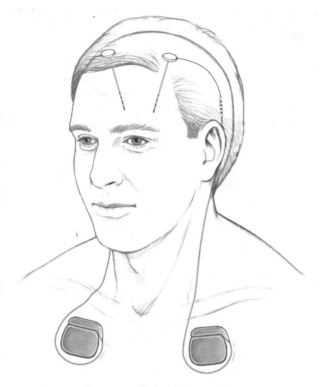

FIGURE 9.2

Bilateral DBS. Note there is also an impulse generator now available that can drive two brain leads from one device (Kinetra®, Medtronic Corporation, Minneapolis, Minnesota).

- Each contact can be activated utilizing monopolar or bipolar stimulation, and multiple settings can be adjusted for individual patient needs.

- These settings include the pulse width (how long the stimulation is), frequency (how often the stimulation is delivered), and amplitude (how much stimulation) of stimulation.

- The DBS lead is placed into a brain target, and is attached to a connector wire and a programmable pulse generator.

- The pulse generator or neurostimulator is placed below the clavicle. The pulse generator is connected to the DBS lead by an attachment wire that travels across the posterior aspect of the neck and skull.

SELECTION OF PATIENTS FOR PARKINSON'S DISEASE, ESSENTIAL TREMOR, AND DYSTONIA SURGERY

Careful patient selection is the first and perhaps the most important step for success of DBS. There are no standardized criteria for choosing candidates, and criteria may differ depending on the targeted symptom or disorder. The next section discusses the important aspects of patient selection that should be considered in PD, essential tremor (ET), dystonia, and OCD/Tourette.

Parkinson's Disease

- PD, which is a slowly progressive neurodegenerative disorder (cardinal manifestations are resting tremor, bradykinesia, rigidity, and gait disorder), presents many challenges for the practitioner who is considering offering DBS.

- There are no set criteria for surgical candidacy, and only recently has a screening questionnaire for this purpose been developed and reported.[2]

  - The Florida Surgical Questionnaire for PD (FLASQ-PD) is a five-section questionnaire that includes: (1) criteria for the diagnosis of "probable" idiopathic PD, (2) potential contraindications to PD surgery, (3) general patient characteristics, (4) favorable/unfavorable characteristics, and (5) medication trial information subscores.

  - The scoring system was designed to assign higher scores to better surgical candidates. The highest/best possible FLASQ-PD score is 34 with 0 "red flags," and the lowest/worse possible FLASQ-PD score is 0 with 8 "red flags." A red flag is a sign or symptom that would automatically put a patient at high risk for a complication of surgery. A score of approximately 25 without red flags indicates a potentially good surgical candidate.

  - This questionnaire can be filled out and scored by a general neurologist. Potential candidates who score well on this questionnaire will then require medical optimization with a movement disorders specialist (if needed), a neurosurgery consultation, a special magnetic resonance image (MRI) for targeting, and a full neuropsychologic evaluation. Some patients may additionally require a speech and swallowing evaluation and psychiatric evaluation for treatment of active affective disorders.

- In general, the best PD surgical candidates have idiopathic PD (not other causes of parkinsonism, which includes other diagnoses such as multiple system atrophy, progressive supranuclear palsy, Lewy body disease, corticobasal ganglionic degeneration), tend to be younger (below age 69, but may be older), have a clear response to medication (at least 30% improvement, but preferably higher), with significant motor fluctuations (e.g., "wearing off" of medications prior to the next dose, "on-off" fluctuations, dyskinesias), and have no or little cognitive dysfunction.

- Perhaps the most controversial aspect of patient selection often involves defining unacceptable cognitive dysfunction, especially since many PD patients suffer from some frontal and memory deficits, but are quite functional in their daily lives. A general rule is that PD patients with a lot of memory or cognitive problems, and those who become disoriented frequently are poor candidates and can be made worse with DBS surgery.

Essential Tremor

- In ET, patients suffer from postural tremor (holding the hands and arms in a fixed position) and action tremor (tremor when they attempt tasks), which often disrupts the simple, but important, daily tasks such as handwriting or drinking.

- ET candidates for DBS must have medication-refractory tremor defined as having failed maximal titrations and preferably combinations of a beta blocker, primidone, and possibly a benzodiazepine. There are other medications that have been found effective in some patients with ET, and these may be tried as well.

- The tremor must be interfering with the quality of life to consider surgery.

- There are no available questionnaires to screen for good ET surgical candidates; however, the same interdisciplinary workup is necessary (as was discussed for PD), and it is important that the tremor be diagnosed correctly as ET can be confused with other tremor subtypes.

  - Again, the most difficult criteria to interpret for the ET surgical candidate is the neuropsychologic screening data, especially since it has recently been appreciated that ET can be associated with frontal lobe and memory dysfunction.

Dystonia

- Other disorders which may be addressed by DBS have been less studied in terms of selection criteria. In general, the best dystonia surgical candidates suffer from generalized disease (i.e., involving multiple body regions), which may or may not be the result of an identified genetic defect.

  - These criteria are generality based on limited experience; however, as more reports of DBS for focal dystonia emerge, the criteria may be expanded.

  - Secondary dystonia, or dystonia due to other causes such as trauma, toxin, birth defect, or metabolic disorder, seems to be less responsive to DBS, although the best surgical target remains to be defined for these cases, and there has been some successes reported.

- The dystonic patients need to fail maximal doses of appropriate medications and preferably combinations of medications including anticholinergics, muscle relaxants, and benzodiazepines, and should also undergo the same workup as for PD patients.

- It is helpful in dystonia if the operation is performed before abnormal joint postures become fixed or contracted.

- Patients with generalized dystonia may be normal on detailed neuropsychologic testing, although recently it has been shown that they may suffer from impairments in complex learning. It remains unknown whether the neuropsychologic profile in dystonia patients affects surgical outcome.

Obsessive-Disorder/Tourette's Syndrome

- DBS for OCD or Tourette's syndrome remains investigational at this time.

- All potential candidates should be refractory to standard medical therapies, and informed consent should be obtained from an institutional review board before offering the procedure.

- The profile of the best candidates with these and similar syndromes remains unknown, although all candidates should undergo the same vigorous testing described above, and should be medication refractory.

Since the optimal dystonia candidate remains to be defined, it is in the best interest of the dystonia patient to seek a medical expert in the area and an experienced center for evaluation. Medication and botulinum toxin refractory cervical dystonia as well as craniofacial dystonia may be addressed by DBS in select cases.

Summary

- There are many characteristics that are important for ensuring the best possible outcomes for DBS (or lesion) surgery in the PD patient.

- In general, the best candidate profiles include (1) idiopathic PD patients who are "young" with little or no discernible cognitive dysfunction and those who (2) have undergone multiple medication trials for refractory symptoms.

- It is preferable to have patients screened and worked up for PD surgery in an experienced and well-staffed multidisciplinary center because of the complex preoperative, intraoperative, and postoperative care required for these patients.[3]

- Choosing essential tremor and dystonia candidates may differ in some respects to PD as response to levodopa is not a criterion.

There are several issues that should be thought through when patients present to your clinic considering DBS (Figure 9.3).

Characteristics of a Candidate for DBS or Lesion Surgery

Age

- There is no lower limit on age.
- Upper limit on age is usually 75–78, but can be modified in select cases (e.g., better physiologic age or good overall health may allow criteria to be more flexible).

One study showed a potential increased surgical risk for cognitive dysfunction above the age of 69.[4]

Diagnosis of Idiopathic PD

- Patient must meet the diagnostic criteria for "probable" idiopathic PD.

- Patients should be excluded from surgery if they have another parkinsonian syndrome (progressive supranuclear palsy; Lewy

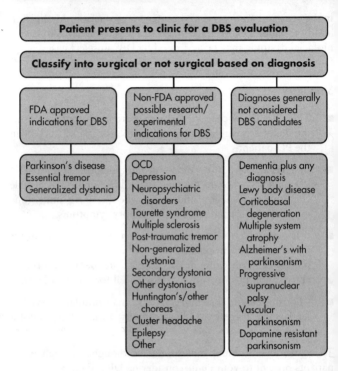

FIGURE 9.3

Current and potential indications for DBS surgery.

body disease; multiple system atrophy, including Shy-Drager syndrome, olivopontocerebellar degeneration, or striatonigral degeneration; corticobasal ganglionic degeneration; vascular parkinsonism; or any other atypical syndrome with parkinsonian features).

On-Off Response to Levodopa

- Patients should be evaluated with the Unified Parkinson's Disease Rating Scale (UPDRS) after abstaining from their medications the night prior to their surgical candidacy workup.

- Section III of the UPDRS (the motor section) should be performed "off" medications and then repeated "on" medications

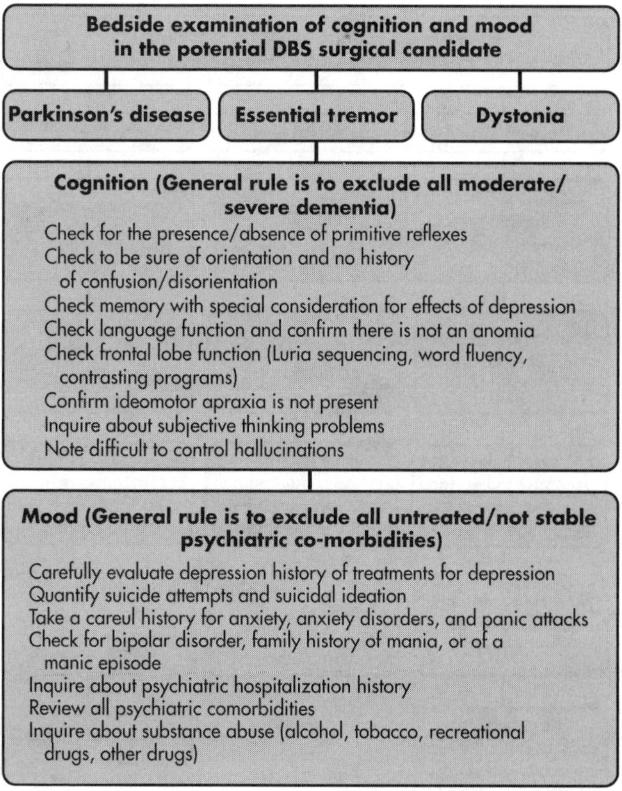

**Bedside examination of cognition and mood
in the potential DBS surgical candidate**

| Parkinson's disease | Essential tremor | Dystonia |

**Cognition (General rule is to exclude all moderate/
severe dementia)**

Check for the presence/absence of primitive reflexes
Check to be sure of orientation and no history
 of confusion/disorientation
Check memory with special consideration for effects of depression
Check language function and confirm there is not an anomia
Check frontal lobe function (Luria sequencing, word fluency,
 contrasting programs)
Confirm ideomotor apraxia is not present
Inquire about subjective thinking problems
Note difficult to control hallucinations

**Mood (General rule is to exclude all untreated/not stable
psychiatric co-morbidities)**

Carefully evaluate depression history of treatments for depression
Quantify suicide attempts and suicidal ideation
Take a careul history for anxiety, anxiety disorders, and panic attacks
Check for bipolar disorder, family history of mania, or of a
 manic episode
Inquire about psychiatric hospitalization history
Review all psychiatric comorbidities
Inquire about substance abuse (alcohol, tobacco, recreational
 drugs, other drugs)

FIGURE 9.4

Evaluation of cognition and mood in a DBS
surgery candidate.

(have patients take their medications and wait for them to
turn "on").

◼ The on-off percentage difference should, in general, exceed
30% to be a reasonable candidate for surgery.

The patient should be examined for nonmotor and motor features during their evaluation with the neurologist (Figures 9.4
and 9.5).

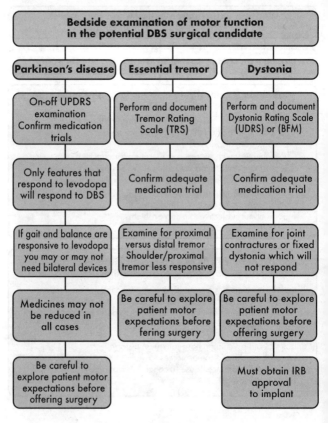

FIGURE 9.5

Motor evaluation of a DBS surgery candidate.

PATIENT EDUCATION: DISCUSSION OF SYMPTOMS THAT RESPOND TO SURGERY

- The results of the on-off evaluation should be discussed in detail with the patient.

- Only "motor" symptoms responding to medications will likely respond to surgery (use the on-off evaluation as the guide to discussion).

- If the patient's gait/balance when optimized on their medication and in their best "on" does not improve, then surgery will likely not help that symptom.

TABLE 9.1
University of Florida Mnemonic Device for Parkinson's Disease Patients Considering DBS[4]

DBS in PD
Does not cure.
Bilateral DBS is often required to improve gait, although sometimes unilateral DBS has a marked effect on walking.
Smoothes out on-off fluctuations.
Improves tremor, stiffness (rigidity), bradykinesia, and dyskinesia in most cases, but may not completely eliminate them.
Never improves symptoms that are unresponsive to your best "on." For example, if gait or balance does not improve with best medication response, it is very unlikely to improve with surgery.
Programming visits are likely to occur many times during the first 6 months, and then follow-up visits as frequently as every 6 months. There will be multiple adjustments in the stimulator and in the medications.
Decreases medications in many, but not all, patients.

- Nonmotor symptoms like depression, anxiety, and quality of life may improve, worsen, or stay the same, but at this time, there are no reliable predictors to reliably discuss with patients.

- It may be useful for the practitioner (both before and after surgery) to have patients study and discuss with him or her a mnemonic device that may help with perceived outcomes[5] (Table 9.1).

CHARACTERISTICS FOR ESSENTIAL TREMOR AND DYSTONIA SURGERY CANDIDATES

- Does not depend on response to levodopa.

- Must be medication refractory (in essential tremor to primidone and beta blockers and in dystonia to carbidopa/levodopa [Sinemet], anticholinergics, muscle relaxants, and benzodiazepines).

Screening Cognitive Dysfunction

- It is important to screen for cognitive dysfunction prior to surgery.

■ There is no clear definition about what is acceptable cognition to become a surgical candidate.

■ Patients who are get lost or become disoriented in general are not good candidates for surgery.

■ Patients with moderate to severe frontal and memory dysfunction may not be good candidates.

■ Patients with a Mini-Mental Status Examination (MMSE) score of <26 or a Mattis Dementia Rating Scale <116 in general may not be good candidates for surgery.

   ■ It is recommended that neuropsychologic testing be done prior to surgery. Table 9.2 lists the typical battery of neuropsychologic tests used in DBS evaluation.

   ■ The neuropsychologic screening may need to be repeated after surgery, especially if cognitive decline is apparent

TABLE 9.2
Neuropsychologic Screening Test for DBS Surgery*

General	Mini-mental Status Exam Mattis Dementia Rating Scale WAIS III (information, vocabulary, matrix)
Learning and Memory	PSAT WAIS III (Digit forward and backward) Hopkins Verbal Learning Task WMS III (stories) Brief Visual Motor Test (BVMT)-R
Language	Wide Range Achievement Test (WRAT) III WTAR Boston Naming Test Controlled Oral Word Association (COWA)
Visuospatial	Judgment of Line Orientation Test (JOLO) Face Recognition Test
Executive	Stroop Test Trail Making Test (Trails A and B) WAIS III (digit symbols)
Mood	Geriatric Depression Scale Beck Depression Scale State-Trait Anxiety Index Visual Analog Mood Scale

* This is a sample screening performed at the University of Florida, but these tests may vary from institution to institution.

(it is useful to have baseline testing for comparison in this situation).

Psychiatric Screening

- There have been increasing reports of psychiatric complications associated with DBS surgery, which include, e.g., depression, depressive symptoms, anxiety, suicide, impulsivity, obsessive-compulsive symptoms, aggression, anger, and mania.

- Although preoperative screening is not required, many centers perform it routinely.

- A preoperative screening with a psychiatrist who can perform a structured clinical interview, make preoperative *Diagnostic and Statistical Manual of Mental Disorders* (DSM) diagnoses, and carefully evaluate depression, anxiety, and mania is useful.

- The psychiatrist may also recommend augmenting the treatment strategy prior to surgery in order to combat depression or anxiety that may impact the intraoperative procedure and/or outcome.

PARKINSON'S DISEASE MEDICATION-REFRACTORY SYMPTOMS AND EXCEPTIONAL CIRCUMSTANCES

- There are circumstances in which a patient may not otherwise be a candidate for PD surgery (e.g., levodopa "on-off" change <30% or cognitive problems), but may have a "special" circumstance (e.g., refractory tremor or dyskinesia).

- Surgery may be considered in the following circumstances, although it may be higher risk:

  - Medication-refractory tremor.

  - Medication-refractory severe dyskinesia.

  - If the patient is on warfarin or other blood thinners. (The patient may have to be hospitalized and use heparin before and after surgery prior to reinstitution of coumadin, depending on individual circumstances.)

  - Medication-refractory and painful dystonia.

MEDICATION TRIALS AND OPTIMIZATION IN PARKINSON'S DISEASE[7]

- A good medication and optimization trial should be implemented before scheduling a PD surgery.

- After a patient undergoes PD surgery, it will be necessary to optimize medications both in preoperative and postoperative management.

- A minority of PD patients will choose not to have surgery after medication optimization (this should be kept in mind when considering "staging" the surgery; i.e., do the right side and see if they need surgery on the left side and vice versa).

- Patients should be tried on maximally tolerated doses of carbidopa/levodopa, dopamine agonists, and dopamine extenders (catecholamine O-methyltransferase [COMT] inhibitors) prior to surgery.

- If patients have dyskinesia, 100 mg one to four times a day of amantadine may be useful. If the dose it too high for an individual patient, a pediatric elixer is available and can be titrated to effect (do not use amantadine with patients who have poor kidney function).

- For patients with nausea as a result of carbidopa/levodopa, the addition of carbidopa 25–100 mg with each dose of carbidopa/levodopa should be considered.

- For patients with medication-refractory tremor, anticholinergics such as trihexyphenidyl or ethopropazine hydrochloride should be tried (watch for, e.g., side effects of mental clouding, urinary retention, confusion).

- For patients who are wearing off between medication doses switching to regular- release carbidopa/levodopa and shortening intervals to every 2, 3, or 4 hours, depending on the situation, should be considered.

- Sudden "offs" may be treated with 1/2–1 tablet of carbidopa/levodopa 25/100 crushed and in orange juice, or alternatively with dissolvable carbidopa/levodopa tablets or apomorphine.

- Dyskinesias and on-off fluctuations can often be managed by changing to regular- release carbidopa/levodopa, decreasing the dose, and moving medication intervals closer together. Further, dopamine agonists (often in lower dose) and dopamine extenders given along with each dose of carbidopa/levodopa may be helpful.

- Rarely, liquid Sinemet may be utilized. If liquid Sinemet is used, patients should crush 10–25/100 tablets and put into 1 L of ginger ale, along with a crushed vitamin C tablet. Every centimeter (or milliliter) equals 1 mg of levodopa. Patients can titrate themselves by sipping the potion all day in an attempt to stay "on" (store away from the sunlight and mix a new batch each day).

MEDICATION TRIALS AND OPTIMIZATION IN ESSENTIAL TREMOR AND DYSTONIA

- ET patients should at a minimum have been tried on maximally tolerated doses of beta blockers and mysoline (if not medically contraindicated).

- Dystonia patients should be tried on maximally tolerated doses and combinations of anticholinergics, muscle relaxants, and benzodiazepines (if not medically contraindicated).

SEEING A MOVEMENT DISORDERS NEUROLOGIST

- Because of the complexity of the screening, it may be beneficial to refer patients to a fellowship-trained movement disorders neurologist who is a member of a multidisciplinary and experienced DBS surgery team.

FACTORS THAT MAY IMPROVE THE SUCCESS OF PD SURGERY

The following list of factors that may improve the success of PD surgery are not evidence based, but are reasonable practice parameters.

- Look for well-trained multidisciplinary experienced DBS teams.

- Look for good (preferably fellowship trained) neurologist-neurosurgeon teams.

- Look for a trained neurologist and/or physiologist in the operating room.

- Look for a full-time DBS programmer.

- Make sure centers perform neuropsychologic and in select cases psychiatric screening.

- Try to choose centers that will partner with you after the surgery so that medication and programming issues can be addressed efficiently. These centers will help to ensure local follow-up for patients traveling to remote centers for their DBS devices.

The use of a DBS multidisciplinary team which many groups believe improve outcomes is summarized in Figure 9.6.

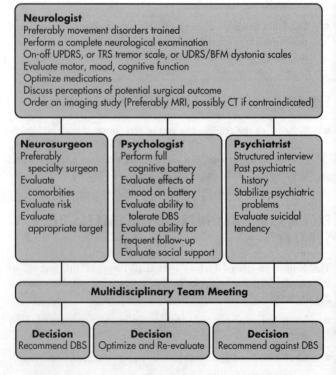

FIGURE 9.6
DBS candidacy evaluation using a multidisciplinary team.

CHOOSING A TYPE (DBS VERSUS LESION THERAPY) AND TARGET (SUBTHALAMIC NUCLEUS VERSUS GLOBUS PALLIDUS) (Figure 9.7)

- DBS is preferred by more patients because it is reversible, and it can be implanted bilaterally without bulbar and cognitive side effects.

- Lesions are preferred by patients who do not want or alternatively cannot have an indwelling piece of hardware. Lesions may also be preferred by those who may not be good candidates for DBS for other reasons (i.e., immunocompromised patients).

- Lesions can be performed bilaterally in the subthalamus and unilaterally in the globus pallidus. Bilateral lesions can be

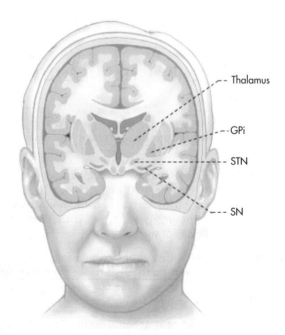

FIGURE 9.7

Usual targets of deep DBS surgery. Shown are the main targets utilized in DBS surgery: thalamus, GPi, and STN (also pictured is the substantia nigra [SN]). The thalamus is a target not commonly employed in PD, but rather for essential tremor. Both DBS and lesion therapy are effective for the treatment of PD.

performed in the pallidum, but carry a high risk of side effects. Thalamic lesions are rarely used in PD because they are limited to tremor control, but bilateral thalamic lesions also may lead to side effects.[8]

■ Lesions can be useful in cases where patients do not have access to DBS programming.

■ The thalamic target is generally effective for tremor, but not the other cardinal manifestations of PD and is therefore not utilized much in PD.

■ Both the globus pallidus (GPi) and the subthalamic nucleus (STN) are very effective targets for DBS therapy.

■ It remains unknown at this time which target is better for which kind of patient (symptom profile).

Going through the thought process of the appropriate target for each patient is important and summarized in Figure 9.8.

DBS TECHNIQUES: INTRAOPERATIVE PLACEMENT OF THE DBS LEAD

■ High-resolution, volumetric MRI is the imaging study of choice both for preoperative screening and for stereotactic targeting.

■ The MRI may be obtained after application of an MRI-compatible stereotactic head ring and localizer on the day of surgery, or the MRI may be obtained nonstereotactically prior to the day of surgery and "fused" to a stereotactic head CT scan on the day of surgery.

■ The latter approach is advantageous because it saves time and minimizes patient discomfort on the day of surgery, and, with appropriate software, the targeting can be performed on the MRI scan in advance of surgery.

■ Stereotactic targeting is a "virtual reality" exercise whereby the target and trajectory within the brain are selected in the *virtual* three-dimensional (3D) space of the volumetric MRI (or, e.g., CT or stereotactic ventriculogram, depending on technique) and translated into the *real* space of the patient's head using stereotactic reference points or "fiducials" that exist in both real and virtual spaces.

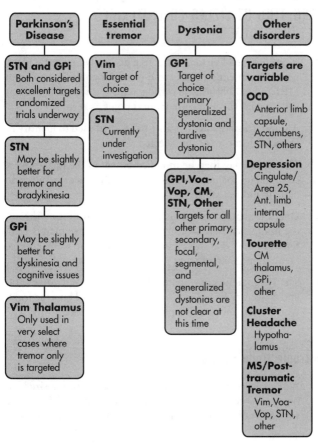

FIGURE 9.8
Choosing a target for DBS surgery.

- In most cases, a stereotactic ring is applied to the patient's head under local anesthesia the day of surgery.

- A CT (or MRI) scan is then obtained with a localizer attached to the ring that allows any point in the volumetric brain image set to be located precisely relative to the position of the ring, which remains in a fixed position relative to the patient's head throughout the procedure.

- If an "image fusion" technique is used, the stereotactic CT is precisely fused to the preoperatively acquired MRI, and targeting is performed on the MR images.

TARGETING UTILIZING COMPUTERIZED METHODOLOGY

- Computerized "virtual" targeting generally begins by identifying the patient's anterior and posterior commissures on the MRI and establishing an orthogonal 3D cartesian coordinate system with the mid commissural point as zero.

- A standard stereotactic brain atlas is then used to identify the expected location of the selected target.

- The target may then be modified based on the images to accommodate for perceived anatomic differences between the patient and the atlas.

- Once the anatomic target is selected, a safe trajectory through the brain is chosen and the "virtual" operative plan is transferred to the "real space" of the patient's head using a stereotactic frame that attaches to the head ring during surgery.

- The stereotactic coordinates that define the operative target and trajectory from the virtual plan are dialed into the frame, which then guides the implantation of electrodes.

Microelectrode Recording

- A 3-cm incision is made and an approximately dime-sized burr hole is placed in the skull at the stereotactically defined entry site (generally frontal, in the region of the coronal suture).

- The lead can either be placed at this time by feeding it through the stereotactic guide and the burr hole to the X, Y, and Z coordinates of the anatomically selected target, or the target can be refined physiologically through the use of microelectrode recording.

- The use of microelectrode recording may minimize the inaccuracy of stereotactic targeting which can be significant and may lead to a suboptimal outcome or even worse, unacceptable side effects.

- If microelectrode recoding is used, the patient is usually kept awake during the operation and minimal to no sedation given (as this may disrupt microelectrode recoding).

- The patient's dopaminergic medications are discontinued 12 hours prior to the operation to improve the chances of picking up abnormal physiologic activity.

- A microelectrode is a recording instrument made of platinum-iridium or tungsten, with a diameter measured in microns that is used to get close to single neurons and record their audible activity and physiologic characteristics (on an oscilloscope).

Techniques to Perform Microelectrode Recording

- The first technique is target verification. A microelectrode may be inserted into a deep brain structure, and if the target or enough of the target is encountered, a DBS lead is placed in this location.

    - This technique, although the least traumatic, may be problematic and lead to potential higher rates of lead misplacement and motor, mood, and cognitive side effects, but this is an issue that is currently under debate.

- A second technique is true physiologic mapping.

    - Physiologic mapping involves identifying the physiology of target and surrounding regions, searching for sensorimotor cells (that respond to movement or touch), identifying borders of the target nucleus with surrounding structures (e.g., optic tract, sensory nucleus, internal capsule), and documenting improvements and side effects.

- The procedure of microelectrode mapping varies somewhat depending on the target. In all cases, however, a 3D picture of the target structure is constructed and compared to standard atlas slices to determine optimal lead positioning.

- Of course, the target in the atlas does not, in general, conform exactly to the same target in a given patient, but the relative sizes and positions of brain structures vary only slightly and the atlas serves as a very useful guide.

- Multipass microelectrode recording, although potentially more accurate than target verification, is more traumatic.

- The third microelectrode recording technique involves the use of five simultaneous electrodes and has been termed the "Ben gun."

    - This approach utilizes stereotactic targeting, physiology, and clinical examination during microstimulation to choose the best location for the final lead placement.

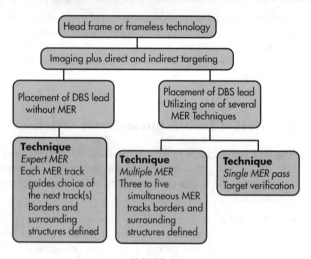

FIGURE 9.9

Techniques that can be utilized for microelectrode recording.

■ The neuropsychologic, mood, and behavioral consequences of single or multiple passes with the microelectrode through the frontal lobes and other subcortical structures is currently being researched.

The techniques that can be utilized for microelectrode recording are summarized in Figure 9.9.

Microelectrode and/or semimicroelectrode recording allow precise physiologic localization of a target region. Each time a new structure is encountered, a different physiologic signature can be decoded (Figure 9.10).

CELLS ENCOUNTERED WHILE MAPPING THE GPi

■ Striatum

■ Low spontaneous discharges 4 Hz

■ Injury discharges

■ Occasionally tonically active cells at 4–6 Hz

■ Globus pallidus externa (GPE)

■ High-frequency discharges (HFDs) (50 ± 21 Hz)

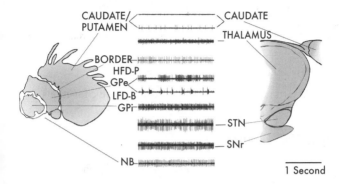

FIGURE 9.10

Example of microelectrode recording in the GPi and STN. (Courtesy of Benjamin Walter, M.D., and Jerry Vitek, M.D., PhD.)

- ■ Separated by pauses (Ps) (HFD-P high-frequency discharge pause cells)
- ■ Ten to 20% of the cells are low frequency P $(18 \pm 12$ Hz)
- ■ May have high-frequency short-duration bursts

■ **GPi**

- ■ High frequency $(82 \pm 24$ Hz)
- ■ HFD but more tonic
- ■ Also, chugging cells—HFDs with pauses that may sound like a chugging train
- ■ 4–6 Hz overt tremor cells can sometimes be heard

■ **Border Cells**

- ■ Frequency (34 ± 19)
- ■ Same as basalis cells, considered aberrantly located basalis cells
- ■ Sound like a motorboat

GPi—Characteristics that Define the Region

- ■ Sensorimotor areas are posterior and lateral.
- ■ They can be identified by passive manipulations.

■   The caudal lateral portions of GPi are movement sensitive.

■   Leg region—medial and dorsal (when compared to arm and face).

■   Jaw-ventral region.

■   Anteromedial—nonmotor associative/limbic functions.

Optic Tract Location

■   Flashing a light into the eyes can give frequency modulation of the background.

■   Can hear the audio signal.

■   Can also microstimulate (see speckles of light in the contralateral visual field).

Internal Capsule

■   Stimulate at 5–40 μA (or higher) and 300 Hz.

■   Stimulation may induce a movement of the limbs or orofacial structures.

MICROELECTRODE LOCALIZATION OF SUBTHALAMUS

■   Depending on where the electrode pass is anterior-posterior will depend on how much thalamus is recorded prior to entering STN. Absence of thalamic recording usually indicates a more anterior trajectory has been chosen.

■   Cell density in the STN is extremely high.

■   Background noise is high and individual cells are difficult to isolate.

■   Single neurons discharge at 20–30 Hz, but most recordings are of multiple cells so the apparent discharge frequency is higher.

■   As the electrode passes through the inferior border of the STN into the substantia nigra (SNr), the discharge pattern changes abruptly. Background noise usually dissipates. Then single neurons with a higher discharge rate of 50–80 Hz (SNr) can be heard.

- Important landmarks—medial border STN is lemniscal (sensory) and the lateral and anterior border STN are corticospinal fibers.

- The medial and lateral borders can be defined by microstimulation- and macrostimulation-evoked sensory and motor responses.

- Unlike the GPi target (where you obtain the posterior and lateral border of the initial plane), the goal of multiple-pass STN mapping is to define the anterior and lateral border.

DBS OR LESION TECHNIQUES: MACROSTIMULATION

- Once the final target coordinates have been chosen (with or without the use of microelectrode recording), the DBS lead is implanted (or alternatively a lesion is placed).

- The final location of the DBS lead may be verified with intraoperative x-rays (fluorography).

- Macrostimulation is then performed by attaching a temporary pulse generator to the DBS electrode and applying current at each of the four electrode contacts in bipolar configurations.

- An intraoperative tester (preferably a neurologist) may rate clinical improvements (tremor, rigidity, bradykinesia, mood changes) or side effects (e.g., muscle contraction due to internal capsule stimulation, paresthesias from stimulation of the sensory thalamus or medial lemniscus, diplopia or visual symptoms from oculomotor or optic tract stimulation, mood changes from stimulation of limbic pathways) to decide if the thresholds for improvement and/or side effects are acceptable.

- The lead may be removed and replaced during this intraoperative session if the intraoperative tester feels the lead is not in an optimal location.

- Adjustments (i.e., moving the lead to a different location) of the lead (intraoperatively) after the first macrostimulation pass may lead to current shunts and consequently mislead the intraoperative tester.

- The neuropsychologic, mood, and behavioral consequences of single or multiple passes with the DBS lead through the frontal lobes and other subcortical structures are unknown.

SECURING THE LEAD AND IMPLANTING GENERATORS

■ After the DBS electrode is implanted at its final location, it is secured to the skull with a specialized plastic burr hole cover (or alternate securing mechanism) and the redundant electrode is buried under the scalp.

■ Under anesthesia, and commonly in a separate, staged procedure, a programmable pulse generator is implanted in a subcutaneous pocket under the clavicle.

■ An extension cable is then tunneled under the skin from the pulse generator to the scalp and connected to the implanted DBS electrode to complete the DBS system.

■ Most centers prefer to wait approximately 30 days before attempting to program the device so that inflammation and brain edema around the DBS electrode has time to resolve.

■ How long it takes for the neuropsychologic, mood, and behavioral consequences resulting from the surgery to resolve remains unknown and under investigation.

DBS PROGRAMMING: GENERAL CONCEPTS

■ After activation, the DBS programmer can telemetrically set the device to one of thousands of different stimulation combinations.

■ The device may be programmed and reprogrammed as many times as is needed.

■ The stimulation parameters therefore can be adjusted to the needs of an individual patient.

■ There may, however, be tradeoffs in programming the stimulator, as the site of optimal motor improvement may cause adverse cognitive or mood side effects and vice versa.

■ It is, therefore, of paramount importance that centers place the devices into an optimal target location. Specifically, DBS leads should be implanted into the sensorimotor territories of the target nuclei (e.g., sensorimotor STN, GPi, thalamus), and care should be taken not to place the lead too close to surrounding anatomy that may result in current spread and side effects.

■ Leads placed in the nuclei but causing current spread into limbic and associative regions may cause further adverse mood and cognitive effects.

■ Teams implanting and programming DBS devices should monitor the short- and long-term motor, mood, cognitive, and behavioral consequences of DBS.

SIMPLE ALGORITHM FOR PROGRAMMING DBS DEVICES IN THE OFFICE

1. Obtain an image and measure placement of the device (CT/MRI or fusion) relative to the anterior commissure, posterior commissure, and midline.

2. Check impedances (>2000 Ω may indicate a connection problem, broken, lead, or lead fracture; <50 Ω may indicate a short).

3. Compare the lead location to standard atlas coordinates (see below) as well as your gross impression as to lead placement.

4. Check impedances of the electrode and perform a battery check.

5. Use the programmer on monopolar for each lead (0, 1, 2, 3) and (frequency 135 Hz; pulse width 60–90 ms) and slowly increase the voltage until you get a side effect (preferably not a transient side effect <30 s). Record both the side effect and the benefit(s) evidenced at each contact.

6. Choose a contact (the best contact) in monopolar to use for chronic DBS (remember that voltage used above 3.6 on the Soletra will dramatically worsen battery life).

7. Try bipolar settings if DBS has too many side effects or if you are not satisfied with the benefit.

8. Slowly decrease the medications and intervals but do not stop them. Look for the best mix of medications and DBS. You may not be able to change many medications with unilateral DBS. Bilateral STN or GPi DBS may require significant medication reductions or changes in medication intervals.

9. Always program patients off medications.

10. For complex patients, after you finish programming, have them take their medications and wait to reexamine in the "on" medication, "on" DBS conditions.

11. Stimulation-induced side effects may require reductions or changes in both medications and stimulation settings.

If there is great difficulty programming a lead, consider referral to an experienced center as the lead may be misplaced.

Figure 9.11 summarizes a simple algorithmic approach to DBS programming:

■   Following initial programming visits, patients should be seen for follow-up programming "off" of medications if they have PD.

■   Be careful programming the device in the first few weeks following implantation as the edema from the lead may lead to difficulties in finding appropriate DBS parameters.

■   Medications in all disorders can be slowly weaned.

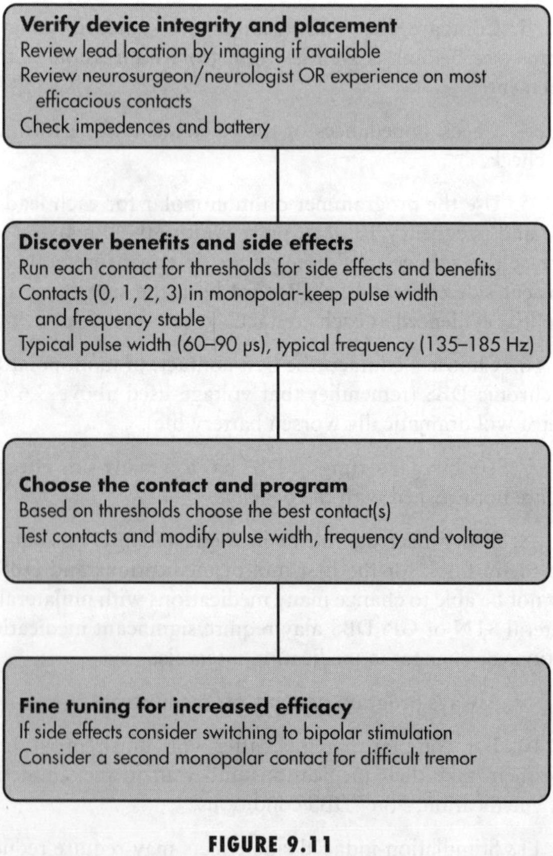

Verify device integrity and placement
Review lead location by imaging if available
Review neurosurgeon/neurologist OR experience on most
    efficacious contacts
Check impedances and battery

Discover benefits and side effects
Run each contact for thresholds for side effects and benefits
Contacts (0, 1, 2, 3) in monopolar-keep pulse width
    and frequency stable
Typical pulse width (60–90 μs), typical frequency (135–185 Hz)

Choose the contact and program
Based on thresholds choose the best contact(s)
Test contacts and modify pulse width, frequency and voltage

Fine tuning for increased efficacy
If side effects consider switching to bipolar stimulation
Consider a second monopolar contact for difficult tremor

FIGURE 9.11
DBS programming algorithm.

- In PD, time between medication intervals may sometimes be lengthened, doses reduced, and in some cases medications discontinued.

- The majority of patients will require a combination of medication and stimulation and will require multiple adjustments over the life of the device.

- One strategy in PD is to increase medication intervals and then on subsequent visits try to discontinue levodopa extenders (such as tolcapone/entacapone) and amantadine and reduce agonists and levodopa (medication doses and intervals should be changed one at a time and slowly, and previous dose and intervals reinstated if worsening occurs).

- The goal of DBS is not medication reduction and medications should be used if symptoms are improved.

- In select cases of essential tremor and dystonia, medication may be discontinued.

- Visits for stimulation and medication adjustments once a month following implantation can be useful for medication and stimulation adjustments.

STANDARD (INDIRECT TARGETING) COORDINATES FOR ESTIMATING LEAD LOCATIONS WHEN LOOKING AT IMAGING (ATLAS APPROXIMATIONS)

- GPi
  - Lateral 20–21.5 mm; 2–3 mm anterior to mid commissural point; 4–5 mm inferior to mid commissural point
- STN
  - Lateral 10–12 mm; 0–2 mm posterior to the mid commissural point; 2–3 mm inferior to mid commissural point

SIDE EFFECTS THAT MAY BE ENCOUNTERED WHILE PROGRAMMING THAT HELP WITH LEAD LOCATION

- STN DBS—eye deviation, mydriasis, and dizziness (too medial), paresthesias (too posterior), motor contraction, dysarthria (too anterior and lateral), conjugate eye deviation (too deep), autonomic features (too medial and anterior).

- STN DBS may lead to hemiballism, and voltage should be set low and increased slightly over a number of weeks (usually improves with good symptomatic benefit).

- GPi DBS—visual symptoms (too deep), motor contraction (too posterior and/or medial).

RISKS OF DBS

- The procedure is expensive, and there are risks beyond the actual surgery including lead fractures, infections, premature battery failure, and the need for frequent reprogramming.

- The surgical risks include infection, hemorrhage, subdural hematoma, stroke, seizure, air embolus, lead misplacement, and hydrocephalus.

- The biggest risk is that the results do not meet the patient's preoperative preconceived result.

- Advantages of the DBS system over lesioning therapy include the ability to perform bilateral procedures without speech and cognitive side effects, reversible effects of stimulation, and the ability to optimize the stimulation parameters for increased benefit.

POSTOPERATIVE DBS URGENCIES AND EMERGENCIES

- A change in skin color over the impulse generator or the lead could signify infection, and patients should go to the hospital immediately for evaluation and/or antibiotics. Infections treated quickly and aggressively may obviate the need for device removal.

- Prolonged fever or drainage from the skin close to the device can also signify infection.

- Persistent confusion, disorientation, or mental status change can indicate infection or other neurologic emergencies.

- Rebound of symptoms can signify lead fractures or battery failure.

- Electric shock-like sensations can signify lead shorts.

- Sudden excessive spending of money, pressured talking, gambling, or grandiose behavior can signify mania.

- Feelings of doom, dysphoria, crying, and loss of energy may signify depression and should be treated quickly and aggressively because of the potentially increased risk of suicide in DBS.[6]

- Tenseness, anxiety, and anger outbursts can all be the result of DBS.

- Persistent postoperative headaches can be a sign of hydrocephalus.

- Postoperative seizures can be a sign of hemorrhage, air, or subdural hematomas and should be followed up with immediate imaging studies.

DBS FAILURES

- Since FDA approval of DBS for PD, ET, and dystonia (humanitarian exemption), there has been a surge in the number of medical centers providing the procedure.

- No uniform consensus has been established for the best screening procedures for DBS.

- An emerging problem in the field of DBS is complications of therapy that require referral to an experienced DBS center for management.

- A recent retrospective analysis of 41 consecutive DBS failures showed that all of the complications in this series were preventable and included difficulties in triage, screening, operative procedure, programming, or medication adjustments.[9]

- Misplaced leads in 19 patients (46%) were one of the most common causes of a poor response to DBS.

- Lead placement has a significant impact on the efficacy of DBS, and it is crucial that centers placing DBS electrodes have the appropriate multidisciplinary teams necessary to evaluate, select, and accurately implant and adjust patients offered this therapy.

REFERENCES

1. Vitek JL, Bakay RA, Hashimoto T, et al. Microelectrode-guided pallidotomy: technical approach and its application in medically intractable Parkinson's disease. J Neurosurg 1998;88(6):1027–1043.

2. Okun MS, Fernandez HH, Pedraza O, et al. Development and initial validation of a screening tool for Parkinson disease surgical candidates. Neurology 2004;63(1):161–163.

3. Krack P, Fraix V, Mendes A, et al. Postoperative management of subthalamic nucleus stimulation for Parkinson's disease. Mov Disord 2002;17(Suppl 3):S188–S197.

4. Saint-Cyr JA, Trepanier LL, Kumar R, et al. Neuropsychological consequences of chronic bilateral stimulation of the subthalamic nucleus in PD. Brain 2000;123 (Pt 10):2091–2108.

5. Okun MS, Foote KD. A mnemonic for Parkinson disease patients considering DBS: a tool to improve perceived outcome of surgery. Neurologist 2004;10(5):290.

6. Okun MS, Green J, Saben R, et al. Mood changes with deep brain stimulation of STN and GPi: results of a pilot study. J Neurol Neurosurg Psychiatry 2003;74(11):1584–1586.

7. Romrell J, Fernandez HH, Okun MS. Rationale for current therapies in Parkinson's disease. Expert Opin Pharmacother 2003;4(10):1747–1761.

8. Okun MS, Vitek JL. Lesion therapy for Parkinson's disease and other movement disorders: update and controversies. Mov Disord 2004;19(4):375–389.

9. Okun MS, Tagliati M, Pourfar M, et al. Management of referred deep brain stimulation failures: a retrospective analysis from 2 movement disorders centers. Arch Neurol 2005;62(8):1250–1255. Epub June 13, 2005.

10

SPEECH AND SWALLOWING THERAPY

SPEECH AND SWALLOWING ABNORMALITIES IN PATIENTS WITH MOVEMENT DISORDERS

Speech and swallowing abnormalities occur frequently in individuals with movement disorders. Evaluation and treatment of motor speech disorders (i.e., dysarthria and apraxia of speech [AOS]) and oropharyngeal dysphagia are typically performed by speech-language pathologists (SLPs). These evaluations and treatments can (1) determine whether speech and swallowing are affected, (2) determine severity and prognosis of speech and swallowing involvement, (3) assist in the formulation of a treatment plan, (4) improve function and quality of life, and (5) assist the medical team in making differential diagnoses. This chapter will summarize procedures utilized by SLPs to evaluate speech and swallowing. The Mayo classification system of motor speech disorders will be introduced with an emphasis on its relevance for physicians and other healthcare providers. Finally, speech and swallowing disorders and their treatment in a variety of movement disorders will be discussed.

EVALUATION OF SPEECH

- SLPs primarily use auditory-perceptual methods to evaluate speech disorders, although instrumental assessment techniques such as direct laryngoscopy, acoustic analysis of speech, and kinematic measurement approaches are becoming increasingly common.

■ A traditional clinical motor speech evaluation consists of four components:

   1. A history

   2. Examination of the speech mechanism with nonspeech activities

   3. Maximum performance testing of the speech mechanism

   4. Evaluation of speech performance during a variety of speaking tasks

Figure 10.1 reviews the components of typical assessment procedures for speech disorders in greater detail.

THE MAYO CLASSIFICATION SYSTEM OF SPEECH DISORDERS

■ Darley et al.[2–4] refined the auditory-perceptual method of classification of speech disorders in a series of seminal works.

■ This classification system, now known as the Mayo system, is based on several premises:

   ■ Speech disorders can be categorized into different types.

   ■ They can be characterized by distinguishable auditory perceptual characteristics.

   ■ They have different underlying pathophysiology associated with different neuromotor deficits.

   ■ Therefore, the Mayo system has value for the localization of neurologic disease and can assist in making differential diagnoses.[5]

   ■ The Mayo system also provides guidance for treatment planning.[6]

■ Table 10.1 details the types of motor speech disorders, their localization, and their neuromotor bases.

BEHAVIORAL TREATMENT OF SPEECH DISORDERS

■ Most treatment approaches for speech abnormalities in patients with movement disorders are presented later in this chapter under the sections on specific medical diagnoses.

History of the speech problem	Examination of the speech mechanism with nonspeech activities	Examination of the speech mechanism with non speech activities	Evaluation of the speech mechanism with speech tasks
Onset and course Insidious or acute, fluctuations over time, effects of medication	**Respiratory mechanism** Observe for posture, breathing at rest, and with physical exertion. Elicitation of brisk sniff and rapid pant determines strength and coordination of the respiratory mechanism	**Respiratory mechanism** Assess range of loudness and maximum loudness during phonation. Measure maximum phonation duration	**Connected speech** Considered the most critical part of the evaluation. Used to determine how components of an individual's speech mechanism work together. Used to assess speech characteristics including rate, intonation, stress, rhythm, and natural-ness. Elicited during histroy or conversation (i.e., "Tell me about your family")
Associated deficits Difficulty with swallowing, cognition, language, and/or changes in affect or emotions, physical function	**Larynx** Laryngeal integrity assessed by eliciting volitional coughs and grunts. Direct visualization of the laynx via flexible fiberoptic endsoscopy orrigid oral laryngoscopy may be necessary in some patients.	**Larynx** Assess vocal quality during 3 seconds of the optimal phonation. Assess pitch range with pitch glide from lowest to highest pitch	
Patient perception Patient describes change in speech and strategies to improve speech		**Velopharynx (VP)** Assess resonance during assimilative nasality task ("Make me a Hong Kong cookie") and during production of a standard sentence ("Buy Bobby a poppy") with the nares open and occluded.	**Repeating words/ sentences:** 1. Snowball 2. Impossibility 3. Catastrophe 4. Please put the groeries in the refrigerator 5. The valuable watch was missing 6. The shipwreck washed up on the shore[102]
Consequences of speech disorder Changes in ability to participate in vocational or social activities	**Velopharynx (VP)** Evaluate VP at rest for symmetry, involuntary movements, or structural abnormalities		
Overall health care Other professionals involved, services provided, current medications, utilization of community resources[5,42]	**Orofacial mechanism (face/lips, jaw, tongue)** Determines symmetry, strength, range of motion, and coordination. Observe for involun-tary movements, structural abnorm-alities, and abnormal posturing[5]	**Orofacial mechanism** Assess alternating motion rate by instructing patients to repeat "puh," "tuh," "kuh" as quickly, precisely, and regularly as they are able. To isolate the tongue for "kuh," have patient put thumb between teeth, and bite down lightly[101]	**Reading a standard passage** Use a passage with knownnumber of words, frequency of sounds, and established rate norms, such as the Grandfather Passage[5] (See Appendix A.)

FIGURE 10.1

Key components of a traditional clinical motor speech evaluation.

Table 10.1
Types of Motor Speech Disorders, Their Localization, and
Their Neuromotor Basis

Type	Localization	Neuromotor basis
Flaccid dysarthria	Lower motor neuron	Weakness
Spastic dysarthria	Bilateral upper motor neuron	Spasticity
Ataxic dysarthria	Cerebellar control circuit	Incoordination
Hypokinetic dysarthria	Basal ganglia control circuit	Rigidity or reduced range of movements
Hyperkinetic dysarthria	Basal ganglia control circuit	Abnormal movements
Mixed dysarthria	More than one	More than one
Apraxia of Speech	Left (dominant) hemisphere	Motor planning/ programming

- Regardless of medical or speech diagnosis, certain therapeutic principals apply:

  - Treatment should be aimed at maximizing intelligibility and naturalness.

  - For maximum benefit, patients and families must be committed to rehabilitation.

  - In many instances, treatment will need to be intensive.

- For further details regarding principles of treatment for motor speech disorders, see Rosenbek and Jones.[7]

EVALUATION OF SWALLOWING

- Swallowing function is usually considered to comprise three stages:

  1. Oral stage

  2. Pharyngeal stage

  3. Esophageal stage

- Assessment and treatment of oral and pharyngeal stages of swallowing are within the scope of practice for SLPs as part of an interdisciplinary team including physicians, surgeons, occupational therapists, dieticians, nurses, dentists, and other health-care professionals, while esophageal dysphagia is managed primarily by physicians (i.e., gastroenterologists).

- Evaluation of oropharyngeal swallowing typically begins with a clinical swallowing evaluation. The traditional components include:

  - A history

  - An oral motor examination, often with sensory testing

  - A physical examination to assess items such as voice quality, strength of cough, and palpation of laryngeal excursion with swallowing

  - Observation of how foods and liquids are swallowed

- Instrumental assessment techniques may also be necessary, such as videofluoroscopic swallowing evaluation (VFSE) and/or fiberoptic endoscopic evaluation of swallowing (FEES), which allow a skilled clinician to:

  - Assess the integrity of the oropharyngeal swallowing mechanism.

  - Establish the biomechanical abnormalities causing dysphagia.

  - Make appropriate recommendations with regard to oral intake, therapeutic intervention, and consultations to other health-care professionals.

- VFSE and FEES also allow for assessment of penetration and aspiration, which are especially critical signs because of their potential negative effects on health.

  - Penetration occurs when material enters the larynx but does not pass into the trachea. Figure 10.2 shows penetration during VFSE.

  - Aspiration occurs when material passes through the larynx and into the trachea. Figure 10.3 shows aspiration during VFSE.

  - Both aspiration and penetration can be measured during VFSE with the penetration-aspiration scale, an eight-point scale to quantitatively measure the depth of airway entry and whether or not the material is expelled.[8]

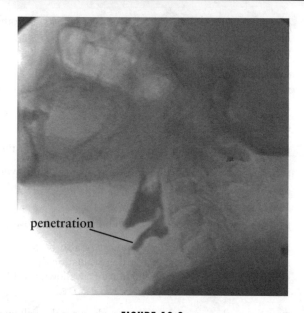

FIGURE 10.2
Penetration, or entry of material into the larynx but not the trachea, is shown during VFSE.

BEHAVIORAL TREATMENT OF SWALLOWING DISORDERS

■ Behavioral treatments for dysphagia in patients with movement disorders are based primarily on the biomechanical abnormalities observed during evaluation. Treatments for dysphagia tend to be less condition specific than those for speech. Therefore, the most common methods are discussed below, and this list will be referenced in subsequent sections. Specific treatment approaches with application to particular patient populations will follow later in this chapter.

■ Regardless of medical diagnosis, if swallowing (1) remains unsafe, (2) inadequate to maintain hydration and nutrition, or (3) requires more effort than the patient can tolerate, a variety of behavioral treatments can be considered.

■ Appropriate behavioral treatments can be most effectively determined with an instrumental assessment of swallowing, which allows for a biomechanical analysis of swallowing to be completed.

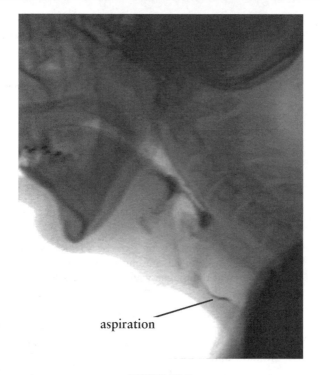

FIGURE 10.3
Aspiration, or entry of material into the trachea, during
VFES is shown.

- Behavioral treatments can be categorized into rehabilitative and compensatory approaches. General behavioral treatments for patients with dysphagia are described below.

- Rehabilitative treatments include the following:

  - *Supraglottic swallow* is an airway protection technique which involves forceful laryngeal adduction followed by a throat clear/cough and a repeated swallow.[9]

  - *Mendelsohn's maneuver* is primarily a technique to prolong upper esophageal sphincter[10] (UES) opening involving holding the larynx for 1–3 seconds in its most anterior-superior position followed by completion of the swallow.[9]

  - *Shaker head raise* is an exercise for increasing UES opening in which a patient lies supine and repetitively raises and lowers his or her head.[11,12]

- *Lee Silverman voice treatment* (LSVT) is a series of maximum performance exercises primarily associated with dysarthria rehabilitation. LSVT may also have a general therapeutic effect on swallowing movements.[13]

- *Expiratory muscle strength training* (EMST) is an exercise which uses a pressure threshold device to overload the muscles of expiration. EMST may have a general therapeutic effect on speech and swallowing movements.[14]

- *Showa's maneuver* requires the forceful elevation of the tongue against the palate followed by a long hard swallow during which the patient is instructed to squeeze all the muscles of the face and neck. This technique appears to influence oral and pharyngeal movements during swallowing.

- *Masako's technique* is an exercise to increase posterior pharyngeal wall movement involving protruding and holding the tongue while executing a forceful dry swallow.[15]

- *Lingual strengthening techniques* include a variety of techniques involving movement of the tongue against resistance, which may improve oral stage function and swallow initiation.[16]

- *Sensory therapies* include stimulation with cold, sour, and electrical current. These treatments may improve oral and pharyngeal stage function.[17,18]

- If rehabilitative treatments are unsuccessful or impractical, a variety of compensatory treatments can be considered.

  - General postural stabilization

  - Postural adjustments to the swallowing mechanism, including the chin tuck and head turn

  - Throat clearing or coughing to clear airway after swallowing

  - Repeated swallows to clear oropharyngeal residue

  - Use of a "liquid wash" to clear oropharyngeal residue

  - Controlling bolus size with instruction or adaptive equipment

  - Smaller, more frequent meals to optimize nutritional intake and swallowing function, especially if swallowing is effortful or causes fatigue

- Eliminating troublesome foods from the diet or preparing them in a softer, moister form

- Dietary supplements

- Timing of eating and drinking to coincide with maximal medication effects

- Thickening liquids and pureeing foods as a last resort

- If rehabilitative and compensatory strategies are inadequate, decisions about enteral nutrition may become necessary.

SPEECH AND SWALLOWING IN PARKINSON'S DISEASE
Speech Disorders

- Hypokinetic dysarthria occurs in most individuals with Parkinson's disease (PD) at some point in the progression of the disease, with approximately 90% of PD patients having dysarthria in some series.[19,20] See Appendix B for a description of the perceptual features of hypokinetic dysarthria.

- Hypokinetic dysarthria may be the presenting symptom of neurologic disease for some individuals with PD.

- The term *hypophonia* is often used to describe the decreased vocal loudness of individuals with PD.

- Inappropriate silences may occur frequently and be associated with difficulty initiating movements for speech production.

- Neurogenic stuttering, consisting most often of sound and word repetitions, may also be observed in some patients with PD.

- Individuals with PD appear to have a perceptual disconnect between their actual loudness level and their own internal perception of loudness.

- When patients have insight into their speech problem, they often describe the presence of a "weak" voice. They may report avoiding social situations that require speech.

- The severity of dysarthria may not correspond to the duration of PD or severity of other motor symptoms.

- Hyperkinetic dysarthria, rather than hypokinetic dysarthria, may also be encountered. This most often occurs in the presence of dyskinesias, particularly after prolonged levodopa therapy.

- Other communication disorders commonly encountered in patients with PD include cognitive impairments, masked facies, and micrographia.

Treatment

- Although a variety of medical and surgical approaches have been attempted to improve the speech of patients with PD, behavioral treatments have shown the most sustained beneficial effect.[21]

- LSVT has a robust literature supporting its beneficial effects and is the treatment of choice for individuals with PD and hypokinetic dysarthria.[22–25]

- Other maximum performance treatments such as EMST may also be beneficial.[26]

- A variety of other behavioral techniques may also be indicated.

    - Rate-control techniques, such as delayed auditory feedback (DAF), pitch-shifted feedback, and pacing boards.

    - Augmentative-alternative communication (AAC) treatment approaches such as the use of voice amplifiers or speech-generating computers may also be appropriate, particularly as dysarthria progresses in severity.

- For many individuals with PD, pharmacologic treatment does not appear to have a significant beneficial impact on speech production, although speech function may be improved in some patients.

- Surgical treatments for PD also do not appear to have a consistent significant benefit for the speech disorders encountered in PD. Although improved speech performance may occur in some patients after surgery, this is not considered an expected outcome. Speech may be unchanged or worsened following surgery.

Swallowing Disorders

- Oropharyngeal dysphagia has been reported in up to 90–100% of people with PD. However, dysphagia is often unrecognized or underestimated by patients.[27-29]

- Oropharyngeal dysphagia may be the initial symptom and a particular pattern of lingual fenestration characterized by repetitive tongue pumping motions is considered a pathognomic sign of PD.[9]

- The severity of dysphagia may not correspond to the duration of PD or severity of other motor symptoms.

- All stages of swallowing function can be affected in patients with PD.

    - Oral stage deficits may include drooling, increased oral transit time, repetitive tongue pumping motions, and premature spillage of the bolus.

    - Pharyngeal stage function may be remarkable for a pharyngeal swallow delay, postswallow pharyngeal residue, penetration, and aspiration.

    - Esophageal stage swallowing problems are also common and most frequently include abnormalities in esophageal motility.

Treatment

- General treatment strategies can be found in the section on Behavioral Treatment of Swallowing Disorders.

- Maximum performance techniques typically used in the rehabilitation of speech disorders in PD such as LSVT and EMST may also improve oropharyngeal swallow function.[13]

- Referral to an occupational therapist may be beneficial to determine the appropriateness of adaptive utensils and equipment to promote independence with meals due to the effect of motor symptoms (i.e., tremor) on self-feeding skills.

- Although dopaminergic medications are not typically associated with significant improvements in swallow function, in some patients these medications may provide benefit. In these select cases, "on" effects can be timed to coincide with meals.

- Surgical treatment of PD does not appear to improve swallowing function for most patients, and postoperative dysphagia has been described in the literature as an adverse event.

- Although dysphagia is common in PD, it rarely is severe enough to require an alternative means of nutritional support.

SPEECH AND SWALLOWING DISORDERS IN MULTIPLE SYSTEM ATROPHY

Speech Disorders

- Dysarthria is a common symptom of multiple system atrophy (MSA) which has been reported in up to a 100% of unselected patients in some studies.[30]

- Dysarthria in MSA is usually more severe than in PD and often emerges earlier in the course of the disease.[5]

- Due to the involvement of multiple brain systems in MSA, the presentation of dysarthria can be expected to be heterogeneous and complex.

- A mixed dysarthria with features of hypokinetic, ataxic, and spastic dysarthria types is described most frequently in patients with MSA.[5] See Appendix B for a description of the perceptual features of these dysarthria types.

  - In patients with prominent features of parkinsonism (i.e., MSA-P or striatonigral degeneration [SND]), features of hypokinetic dysarthria may be expected to predominate.

  - In patients with prominent features of cerebellar dysfunction (i.e., MSA-C or olivopontocerebellar atrophy [OPCA]), features of ataxic dysarthria may be most notable.

  - In patients with prominent features of autonomic failure (i.e., Shy-Drager syndrome), ataxic, hypokinetic, and spastic dysarthria types, alone on in combination, have been described.[31]

- Stridor may occur in patients with MSA. This may result in respiratory comprise and even may necessitate a tracheostomy in severe cases. Stridor in MSA has usually been attributed to vocal cord paralysis, but some data suggest the cause is laryngeal-pharyngeal dystonia.[32]

Treatment

- Some data suggest patients with MSA may benefit from LSVT.[33]

- Other maximum performance treatments such as EMST may be a sensible approach in some patients.

Swallowing Disorders

- Dysphagia is a well-known symptom of MSA.

- Dysphagia is often more severe in MSA than in PD.[34]

- Results from VFSE in patients with MSA reveal both oral and pharyngeal stage deficits.

  - Oral stage dysphagia in patients with MSA is often present even in the early stage of the disease and may become severely involved with disease progression. Oral deficits may include difficulty with holding and transporting the bolus.

  - Pharyngeal stage function may also be impaired, but much less so than the oral stage, especially early in the disease. Pharyngeal deficits may include decreased pharyngeal clearance, reduced laryngeal elevation, and incomplete relaxation of the upper esophageal sphincter.[35,36]

- Not surprisingly, dysphagia has also been reported in the literature, which uses the terminology SND, OPCA, and Shy-Drager syndrome (SDS), although it has received little systematic attention.

  - Dysphagia has been reported in 44% of patients with SND and has been described infrequently as the initial symptom.[37,38]

  - In patients with OPCA, dysphagia has been reported in 24–33% of cases and has been described infrequently as the initial symptom.[39]

  - Dysphagia in SDS has received little attention, and it can be hypothesized that oropharyngeal dysphagia may be relatively uncommon in "pure" autonomic failure. Of course, with disease progression and the additional involvement of the extrapyramidal and cerebellar systems, oropharyngeal dysphagia becomes increasingly likely.

Treatment

- General treatment strategies can be found in the section on Behavioral Treatment of Swallowing Disorders.

- Maximum performance techniques such as LSVT and EMST may benefit oropharyngeal swallow function in MSA.

SPEECH AND SWALLOWING IN PROGRESSIVE SUPRANUCLEAR PALSY

Speech Disorders

- Dysarthria is common in patients with progressive supranuclear palsy (PSP). Some series of unselected patients demonstrate the presence of dysarthria in 70–100% of cases.[19,40,41]

- The dysarthria of PSP is a mixed dysarthria with features of hypokinetic, spastic, and ataxic dysarthria types.[5,30] Appendix B details the perceptual features of these dysarthria types.

- Recognizing the presence of a mixed dysarthria in PSP can help to distinguish it from PD.

- Dysarthria in PSP occurs early, often within the first 2 years of the disease.[5]

- Dysarthria is more frequently an initial symptom of neurologic disease in PSP than with PD.[5,19]

- Dysarthria may be severe, even relatively early in the disease. Anarthria or mutism may be exhibited in the later stages of the disease.[42]

- Cognitive-linguistic deficits and other problems which affect communication, such as apathy and disinhibition, may also be present.

Treatment

- Although the data are limited, maximum performance treatments such as LSVT or EMST may be beneficial in the treatment of dysarthria in PSP.[33] This approach may be most sensible when prominent features of hypokinetic and ataxic dysarthria are present.

- DAF has been reported to slow speech rate, increase vocal intensity, and improve intelligibility in PSP.[43]

- The rapid nature of decline in patients with PSP and the frequent cognitive deficits are negative prognostic indicators for treatment. Thus, speech treatments in PSP may be more effective if implemented early in the course of the disease before speech and cognition become severely involved.

Swallowing Disorders

- When swallowing function has been assessed with VFSE, dysphagia has been reported in over 95% of patients with PSP.[44]

- In contrast to patients with PD, individuals with PSP and dysphagia are often aware of their difficulty swallowing, even when they present with cognitive impairments.[19]

- The onset of swallowing difficulties in individuals with PSP may be a negative prognostic indicator for survival.[19,40]

Treatment

- General treatment strategies can be found in the section on Behavioral Treatment of Swallowing Disorders.

- Maximum performance techniques such as LSVT and EMST may benefit oropharyngeal swallow function in patients with PSP

SPEECH AND SWALLOWING IN CORTICOBASAL GANGLIONIC DEGENERATION

Speech Disorders

- The frequency of dysarthria in corticobasal ganglionic degeneration (CBD) has been reported as high as 85%.[45]

- Hypokinetic, spastic, and ataxic dysarthria types, either in isolation or presenting as a mixed dysarthria, occur most frequently.[5,45] Appendix B details the perceptual features of these dysarthria types.

- Dysarthria in CBD may be less severe than other motor impairments.[46]

- AOS has also been reported in cases of CBD[5,47,48] and may be the earliest symptom.[5,49–52] The presence of AOS can be important to differential diagnosis. See Appendix B for a description of the perceptual features of AOS.

- Although rare, the degenerative nature of CBD may eventually lead to the complete inability to produce speech.[53-55]

- Cognitive-linguistic impairments, including aphasia, often coexist with speech disorders in CBD.[4]

Treatment

- Maximum performance treatments such as LSVT or EMST may be sensible when prominent features of hypokinetic and ataxic dysarthria are present.

- Additional targets for treatment of dysarthria in CBD may include:

  - The use of compensatory strategies to increase speech intelligibility, such as reducing the rate of speech, using an alphabet card to identify the first letter of a word, or saying something in a different way when misunderstood.

  - Training the individual and communication partners to use compensatory strategies to achieve successful communication.[56]

- Treatment of AOS with intensive drill of sounds, syllables, words, and phrases may be also useful.

- Advance planning for the acquisition and use of an AAC device is recommended, particularly when cognitive and language skills are relatively intact.[42,57]

Swallowing Disorders

- Swallowing disorders may occur in CBD.

- No distinctive pattern of swallowing difficulty has been reported in patients with CBD.

- The onset of swallowing difficulties in individuals with CBD may be a negative prognostic indicator for survival.[19,40]

Treatment

- General treatment strategies can be found in the section on Behavioral Treatment of Swallowing Disorders.

- Maximum performance techniques such as LSVT and EMST may benefit oropharyngeal swallow function in patients with CBD.

SPEECH AND SWALLOWING IN SYNDROMES OF PROGRESSIVE ATAXIA

Speech Disorders

- Dysarthria is a common symptom in syndromes of progressive ataxia.

- Ataxic dysarthria is the dysarthria type most frequently associated with these conditions. See Appendix B for a description of the perceptual features of ataxic dysarthria.

- Mixed dysarthria may also be encountered when neurologic involvement is not restricted to the cerebellum. A description of the perceptual features of the following dysarthria types may be found in Appendix B.

  - Dysarthria in the spinocerebellar ataxias such as Friedreich's ataxia may present with components of ataxia and spasticity.[5,30]

  - Mixed dysarthria with features of ataxic, hypokinetic, spastic, and flaccid dysarthria types may be encountered in patients with OPCA (see the section on Multiple System Atrophy for further details).[5,30]

Treatment

- The treatment literature associated with dysarthria in syndromes of progressive ataxia is noticeably sparse.

- The literature on treatment of patients with ataxic dysarthria due to a variety of etiologies may provide guidance.

  - Rate-control strategies can be beneficial in improving intelligibility in patients with ataxic dysarthria.[58] Appropriate strategies may include DAF or use of a pacing board.

  - Maximum performance treatments, such as LSVT and EMST, may have benefit in patients with ataxic dysarthria.[59,60]

Swallowing Disorders

- Dysphagia appears to occur less frequently than dysarthria in patients with progressive ataxia.

- However, VFSE results have shown oral and pharyngeal stage dysphagia, including premature spillage of the bolus, piecemeal deglutition, pharyngeal residue, and aspiration.[61]

- A likely explanation for dysphagic signs is discoordination of oral, pharyngeal, and respiratory movements.

Treatment

- General treatment strategies can be found in the section on Behavioral Treatment of Swallowing Disorders.

- Dietary modifications such as thickened liquids and therapeutic techniques such as the chin tuck and the supraglottic swallow have been reported to be beneficial in preventing aspiration in patients with degenerative ataxia.[61]

SPEECH AND SWALLOWING IN HUNTINGTON'S DISEASE[62]

Speech Disorders

- The chorea of Huntington's disease (HD) also manifests itself in the speech mechanism and results in a hyperkinetic dysarthria. The perceptual features of hyperkinetic dysarthria in chorea are shown in Appendix B.

- Dementia in HD may result in a variety of cognitive-linguistic impairments which have a negative influence on communication.[56]

Treatment

- Yorkston et al. recommend a treatment approach for patients with HD depending on the severity of their dysarthria and coexisting cognitive-linguistic deficits.[56]

  - In patients with mild dysarthria, drills to target prosody, techniques to reduce hyperkinesias in the larynx, and rate-control activities may be beneficial.

  - In patients with moderate dysarthria, behavioral techniques used in patients with mild dysarthria may continue, with the addition of patient and family training for the use of strategies to address communication breakdowns.

■ In patients with HD and severe dysarthria, speech may no longer be understandable. Therapy may focus on techniques such as natural speech with supportive partners, alphabet boards, calendars and memory aids, making choices, yes/no questions, and conversation starters.

Swallowing Disorders

■ In patients with HD who have primarily hyperkinetic symptoms, swallowing difficulties may include uncontrolled tachyphagia, darting lingual chorea, uninhibited swallow initiation, and impaired inhibition of respiration with swallowing (i.e., respiratory chorea).[63,64]

■ Tachyphagia, or rapid uncontrolled swallowing, occurs often in patients with HD and hyperkinetic symptoms.[63,64]

■ In patients with HD who have primarily symptoms of rigidity and bradykinesia, dysphagia is characterized by mandibular rigidity, inefficient mastication, and slow oral transit.

■ Postswallow vallecular residue occurs frequently in patients with HD.[63,64]

■ Laryngeal penetration and aspiration occur infrequently in patients with HD with hyperkinetic symptoms, but are more frequently reported in patients with prominent rigidity and bradykinesia.[63,64]

■ Esophageal dysphagia occurs relatively infrequently, but eructation (excessive belching), aerophagia (swallowing of air), vomiting, and esophageal dysmotility have been noted in some patients.[64]

Treatment

■ General treatment strategies can be found in the section on Behavioral Treatment of Swallowing Disorders.

■ Management approaches often used in patients with HD and dysphagia include postural and position changes, assistive devices, supervision with meals to control rate of consumption and bolus size, dietary changes, and the use of tube feeding.[56]

■ Bracing by having the patient rest their head against a wall or other supportive surface may aid swallowing during the early stage of the disease.

- Successful implementation of these approaches generally requires a great deal of caregiver assistance owing to the cognitive deficits in patients with HD, but they have been reported to have considerable benefit.[65]

- Patients with HD are at increased nutritional risk because of a multitude of factors which include dysphagia, difficulty with food preparation due to chorea and cognitive deficits, impaired self-feeding skills, and increased calorie consumption due to chorea. Dietary supplements and consultations with dieticians may be beneficial in patients with HD.[66]

SPEECH AND SWALLOWING IN WILSON'S DISEASE

Speech Disorders

- Dysarthria occurs commonly in patients with Wilson's disease (WD)[5] and has been reported in over 90% of unselected patients with neurologic manifestations of the disease.[67,68]

- WD is most commonly associated with a mixed dysarthria with features of hypokinetic, spastic, and ataxic dysarthria types.[5] Appendix B details the perceptual features of these dysarthria types.

- Dysarthria has been described to be the most frequent neurologic manifestation of WD.[69]

- Dysarthria may be the presenting symptom of WD.[67]

- Lingual abnormalities such as tremor, involuntary transverse and bilateral movements at rest and with action, and protrusion of the tongue have been described in select cases of WD.[70-72]

- Speech involvement in WD may be complicated by coexisting dementia.

Treatment

- Very little data on the behavioral treatment of dysarthria in WD are available, although the benefit of speech therapy has been described.[1]

- Although pharmacologic treatment with D-penicillamine (with or without zinc sulfate) has been shown to improve many neurologic symptoms of WD, dysarthria may be resistant to this treatment.[73]

- Improvement or elimination of dysarthria following liver transplantation has been described.[68]

Swallowing Disorders

- Dysphagia in WD has received little attention, although swallowing difficulties including drooling may occur.[5] Dysphagia appears to be a less frequent neurologic manifestation of the disease than dysarthria.

- Aspiration may be expected as disease severity increases.

- Pharyngeal and esophageal dysmotility have also been reported.[10,74]

- Sialorrhea, or an excessive secretion of saliva, has also been reported in some cases.[68] This problem is likely related to oropharyngeal dysphagia and decreased frequency of swallowing rather than a true excess in the production of saliva.

Treatment

- General treatment strategies can be found in the section on Behavioral Treatment of Swallowing Disorders.

- The effect of dietary changes, pharmacologic treatment, and liver transplantation on swallowing has received little attention.

SPEECH AND SWALLOWING DISORDERS IN DYSTONIA

Speech Disorders

- When the locus of dystonia targets any of the components of the speech mechanism, hyperkinetic dysarthria may result. See Appendix B for a description of the perceptual features of the hyperkinetic dysarthria associated with dystonia.

  - *Generalized dystonia* may negatively affect respiratory function and be associated with decreased speech intelligibility.[75]

  - *Neck dystonia* (*cervical dystonia* or *spasmodic torticollis*) may have a negative influence on laryngeal function, with lower habitual pitch, restricted pitch range, and decreased phonatory reaction time being described in the literature.[76] Speech differences in neck dystonia are likely due to the effect of postural abnormalities on speech muscle activity and/or changes in the shape of the vocal tract.[5]

- *Laryngeal dystonia* or *spasmodic dysphonia* (SD)[50] (*adductor, abductor,* or *mixed* types) results in prominent laryngeal abnormalities. Adductor SD, the most common type, results in a strained, strangled vocal quality, while abductor SD presents with a voice that is intermittently breathy or aphonic.[5]

- *Mouth and face dystonia* or *oromandibular dystonia* (OMD) may involve the masticatory, lower facial, and tongue muscles in a variety of combinations. When coupled with blepharospasm, this condition is often known as *Meige's syndrome* or *Brueghel's syndrome*. OMD can severely disrupt function of the orofacial mechanism. Speech in OMD has been described as having imprecise consonants, a slow rate, inappropriate pauses, and abnormalities in stress.[77,78]

- *Lingual dystonia* may also occur in isolation, although this is rare. This has been described as unilateral tongue puckering, ridging, and bulging.[79] Lingual dystonia with tongue protrusion in isolation[80] and combined with OMD has also been reported.[81] Lingual dystonia frequently causes dysarthria owing to involvement of the orofacial mechanism.[81] Lingual dystonia coupled with palatal dystonia may also occur in rare cases.[82] In a case such as this, involvement of both the orofacial mechanism and the velopharynx during speech may be expected.

- *Jaw dystonia* can result in either jaw-opening or jaw-closing OMD. Open-jaw dystonia has been reported to be associated with cervical dystonia in some patients.[83,84] Either jaw-opening or jaw-closing OMD can be expected to disrupt the orofacial mechanism component of speech production and the presence of speech difficulties has been reported in patients with this condition.[83,84]

- In dystonias that are considered focal, there may be more widespread involvement than expected. For example, respiratory involvement has been described in patients with cervical dystonia and blepharospasm.[85] Dystonia of the soft palate has been reported in a high percentage of cases with laryngeal involvement (SD or essential voice tremor).[86]

Treatment

- Sensory tricks (geste anatgoniste) such as a light touch to the affected area may also be beneficial for the speech of many patients with dystonia.[5]

- The use of a bite block, a custom fitted prosthesis placed between the lateral upper and lower teeth, has been reported to be beneficial in patients with OMD. Such a device may help to inhibit jaw movements during speech.[87,88]

- The most widely used and accepted therapy for dystonia is local intramuscular injections of botulinum toxin A (BTX), which may have a beneficial influence on speech.[12,89,90]

- Lesion surgery and deep brain stimulation (DBS) are being increasingly used in the management of dystonia. The effects of surgical treatments on speech function are largely unexplored. Dysarthria may occur due to stimulation-related muscle contractions in patients with dystonia treated with DBS.[91]

Swallowing Disorders

- When the locus of dystonia targets any of the components of the swallowing mechanism, dysphagia may result.

  - *Generalized dystonia* may be associated with dysphagia. Coordination of respiration with swallowing may be more difficult in patients with respiratory involvement.

  - *Neck dystonia* (*cervical dystonia* or *spasmodic torticollis*) has been reported to be associated with dysphagia in approximately 50% of unselected patients is some series. Most frequent swallowing abnormalities include a delay in swallow initiation and vallecular residue.[92]

  - *Laryngeal dystonia* or *spasmodic dysphonia*[50] (*adductor, abductor,* or *mixed* types) may result in complaints of dysphagia, but swallowing is usually relatively preserved in comparison to speech deficits.

  - *Mouth and face dystonia* or *oromandibular dystonia* (OMD) (also known as *Meige's syndrome* or *Brueghel's syndrome*) may have a negative effect on swallow function. In a series of unselected patients, 90% presented with swallowing abnormalities which included premature spillage of the bolus and vallecular residue.[93] Other swallowing abnormalities in OMD may include chewing difficulties and other deficits in oral preparation of the bolus.[94]

- *Lingual dystonia* often results in dysphagia. In patients with tongue protrusion lingual dystonia with or without OMD, biting of the tongue and pushing food out of the oral cavity with the tongue has been described.[81]

- *Jaw dystonia* may result in a variety of oral and pharyngeal stage deficits which can be severe.

Treatment

- General treatment strategies can be found in the section on Behavioral Treatment of Swallowing Disorders.

- Dysphagia may occur or be exacerbated by treatments such as BTX injections[95] or selective denervation.[96]

- Lesion surgery and DBS are being increasingly used in the management of dystonia. The effects of surgical treatments on swallowing function are largely unexplored. Dysphagia may occur due to stimulation-related muscle contractions in patients with dystonia treated with DBS.[91]

SPEECH AND SWALLOWING DISORDERS IN TARDIVE DYSKINESIA

Speech Disorders

- Hyperkinetic dysarthria is the dysarthria type associated with tardive dyskinesia (TD).[5]

- Dysarthria in TD is most often due to orobuccal and lingual dyskinesias, but laryngeal and respiratory dyskinesias have also been reported.[5,97–99]

- Hyperkinetic dysarthria may also be the presenting symptom of TD.[99]

Treatment

Medical management of TD appears to be the most appropriate treatment for dysarthria associated with this condition.

■ The literature on behavioral treatments for TD is very limited. Treatments for patients with hyperkinetic dysarthria associated with other etiologies may be appropriate including postural adjustments and the use of a bite block.

Swallowing Disorders

■ Dysphagia in TD most commonly consists of difficulty containing foods and liquids in the mouth, as well as inefficient bolus formation and movement.

■ Coordination of oral and pharyngeal swallowing may result in delayed initiation of the swallow, postswallow pharyngeal residue, and aspiration.

■ Dysphagia can be severe enough to cause weight loss.[100]

Treatment

■ General treatment strategies can be found in the section on Behavioral Treatment of Swallowing Disorders.

■ Medical management of TD appears to be the most appropriate treatment for dysphagia associated with this condition.

REFERENCES

1. Day LS, Parnell MM. Ten-year study of a Wilson's disease dysarthric. J Commun Disord 1987;20(3):207–218.
2. Darley FL, Aronson AE, Brown JR. Motor Speech Disorders. Philadelphia: Saunders, 1975.
3. Darley FL, Aronson AE, Brown JR. Differential diagnostic patterns of dysarthria. J Speech Hear Res 1969;12:249–269.
4. Darley FL, Aronson AE, Brown JR. Cluster of deviant speech dimensions in the dysarthrias. J Speech Hear Res 1969;12:462–496.
5. Duffy JR. Motor Speech Disorders: Substrates, Differential Diagnosis, and Management. 2nd ed. St. Louis: Elsevier, 2005.
6. Duffy JR. Pearls of wisdom—Darley, Aronson, and Brown and the classification of the dysarthrias. Perspect Neurophysiol Neurogenic Speech Language Disord 2005;15(3):24–27.
7. Rosenbek JC, Jones HN. Principles of treatment for sensorimotor speech disorders. In: McNeil MR, ed. Clinical Management of Sensorimotor Speech Disorders. 2nd ed. New York: Thieme. In press.
8. Rosenbek JC, Robbins J, Roecker EB, et al. A penetration-aspiration scale. Dysphagia 1996;11:93–98.

9. Logemann JA. Evaluation and Treatment of Swallowing Disorders. 2nd ed. Austin, TX: PRO-ED, 998.

10. Gulyas AE, Salazar-Grueso EF. Pharyngeal dysmotility in a patient with Wilson's disease. Dysphagia 1988;2(4):230–234.

11. Shaker R, Easterling C, Kern M, et al. Rehabilitation of swallowing by exercise in tube-fed patients with pharyngeal dysphagia secondary to abnormal UES opening. Gastroenterology 2002;122(5): 1314–1321.

12. Shaker R, Kern M, Bardan E, et al. Augmentation of deglutitive upper esophageal sphincter opening in the elderly by exercise. Am J Physiol 1997;272(6 Part 1):G1518–1522.

13. Sharkawi AE, Ramig L, Logemann JA, et al. Swallowing and voice effects of Lee Silverman Voice Treatment (LSVT[R]): A pilot study. J Neurol Neurosurg Psychiatry 2002;72:31–36.

14. Kim J, Sapienza CM. Implications of expiratory muscle strength training for rehabilitation of the elderly: Tutorial. J Rehab Res Dev 2005;42(2):211.

15. Fujiu M, Logemann JA. Effect of a tongue-holding maneuver on posterior pharyngeal wall movement during deglutition. Am J Speech Lang Pathol 1996;5:23–30.

16. Robbins J, Gangnon RE, Theis SM, et al. The effects of lingual exercise on swallowing in older adults. J Am Geriatr Soc 2005; 53(9):1483–1489.

17. Rosenbek JC, Jones HN. Sensorische behandlung oropharyngealer dysphagien bei erwachsenen [Sensory therapies for orohoryngeal dysphagia in adults]. In: Stanschus S, ed. Rehabilitation von Dysphagien. Idstein, Germany: Schulz-Kirchner Verlag, 2006.

18. Hamdy S, Aziz Q, Rothwell JC, et al. Recovery of swallowing after dysphagic stroke relates to functional reorganization in the intact motor cortex. Gastroenterology 1998;115:1104–1112.

19. M.ller J, Wenning GK, Verny N, et al. Progression of dysarthria and dysphagia in postmortem confined parkinsonian disorders. Arch Neurol 2001;58:259–264.

20. Logemann JA, Fisher HB, Boshes B, Blonsky ER. Frequency and cooccurrence of vocal tract dysfunctions in the speech of a large sample of Parkinson patients. J Speech Hear Disorders 1978;43(1): 47–57.

21. Merati AL, Heman-Ackah YD, Abaza M, et al. Common movement disorders affecting the larynx: a report from the neurolaryngology committee of the AAO-HNS. Otolaryngol Head Neck Surg 2005;133(5):654–665.

22. Ramig LO, Countryman S, Thompson LL, Horii Y. Comparison of two forms of intensive speech treatment for Parkinson disease. J Speech Hearing Res 1995;38(6):1232–1235.

23. Ramig LO, Countryman S, Thompson L, Horii Y. Comparison of two forms of intensive speech treatment for Parkinson disease. J Speech Hearing Res 1993;38(5):1232–1251.

24. Ramig LO, Countryman S, O'Brien C, et al. Intensive speech treatment for patients with Parkinson's disease: short- and long-term comparison of two techniques. Neurology 1996;47(6):1496–1504.

25. Ramig LO. Voice treatment for patients with Parkinson's disease: development of an approach and preliminary efficacy data. J Med Speech Lang Pathol 1994;2(3):191–209.

26. Saleem AF, Sapienza CM, Rosenbek JC, et al. The effects of expiratory muscle strength training program on pharyngeal swallowing in patients with idiopathic Parkinson's disease. Talk presented at the 57th Annual Meeting of the American Academy of Neurology, Miami, FL, 2005.

27. Leopold NA, Kagel MC. Dysphagia in progressive supranuclear palsy: Radiologic features. Dysphagia 1997;12:140–143.

28. Leopold NA, Kagel MC. Prepharyngeal dysphagia in Parkinson's disease. Dysphagia 1996;11(1):14–22.

29. Robbins JA, Logemann JA, Kirshner HS. Swallowing and speech production in Parkinson's disease. Ann Neurol 1986;19(3):283–287.

30. Kluin KJ, L. FM, Berent S, Gilman S. Perceptual analysis of speech disorders in progressive supranuclear palsy. Neurology 1993;43:563–566.

31. Linebaugh C. The dysarthrias of Shy-Drager syndrome. J Speech Hear Disord 1979;44(1):55–60.

32. Merlo IM, Occhini A, Pacchetti C, Alfonsi E. Not paralysis, but dystonia causes stridor in multiple system atrophy. Neurology 2002;58(4):649–652.

33. Countryman S, Ramig LO. Speech and voice deficits in Parkinsonian plus syndromes: can they be treated? J Med Speech Lang Pathol 1994;2:211–225.

34. Wenning GK, Quinn NP. Parkinsonism. Multiple system atrophy. Baillieres Clin Neurol 1997;6(1):187–204.

35. Higo R, Tayama N, Watanabe T, et al. Videofluoroscopic and manometric evaluation of swallowing function in patients with multiple system atrophy. Ann Otol Rhinol Laryngol 2003;112(7):630–636.

36. Higo R, Nito T, Tayama N. Swallowing function in patients with multiple-system atrophy with a clinical predominance of cerebellar symptoms (MSA-C). Eur Arch Otorhinolaryngol 2005;262(8):646–650.

37. Gouider-Khouja N, Vidailhet M, Bonnet AM, et al. "Pure" striatonigral degeneration and Parkinson's disease: a comparative clinical study. Mov Disord 1995;10(3):288–294.

38. Kurihara K, Kita K, Hirayama K, et al. Dysphagia in olivopontocerebellar atrophy. [Article in Japanese]. Rinsho Shinkeigaku 1990;30(2):146–150.

39. Berciano J. Olivopontocerebellar atrophy. A review of 117 cases. J Neurol Sci 1982;53(2):253–272.

40. Nath U, Ben-Shlomo Y, Thomson RG, et al. Clinical features and natural history of progressive supranuclear palsy: a clinical cohort study. Neurology 2003;60(6):910–916.

41. Diroma C, Dell'Aquila C, Fraddosio A, et al. Natural history and clinical features of progressive supranuclear palsy: a clinical study. Neurol Sci 2003;24(3):176–177.

42. Yorkston KM, Beukelman DR, Strand EA, Bell KR. Management of Motor Speech Disorders in Children and Adults. 2nd ed. Austin, TX: PRO-ED, 1999.

43. Hanson WR, Metter EJ. DAF as instrumental treatment for dysarthria in progressive supranuclear palsy: a case report. J Speech Hearing Dis 1980;45:268–276.

44. Litvan I, Sastry N, Sonies BC. Characterizing swallowing abnormalities in progressive supranuclear palsy. Neurology 1997;48:1654–1662.

45. Ozsancak C, Auzou P, Jan M, et al. The place of perceptual analysis of dysarthria in the differential diagnosis of corticobasal degeneration and Parkinson's disease. J Neurol 2006;253:92–97.

46. Frattali CM, Sonies BC. Speech and swallowing disturbances in corticobasal degeneration. In: Litvan I, Goetz CG, Lang AE, eds. Corticobasal Degeneration Advances in Neurology. Philadelphia: Lippincott Williams & Wilkins, 2000:153–160.

47. Kertesz A. Pick complex: an integrative approach to frontotemporal dementia: primary progressive aphasia, corticobasal degeneration, and progressive supranuclear palsy. Neurology 2003;9(6):311–317.

48. Frattali CM, Grafman J, Patronas N, et al. Language disturbances in corticobasal degeneration. Neurology 2000;54(4):990–995.

49. Rosenfield DB, Bogatka NS, Viswanath AE, et al. Speech apraxia in cortical-basal ganglionic degeneration [abst]. Ann Neurol 1991; 30:296–297.

50. Gibb WRG, Luthert PJ, Marsden CD. Corticobasal degeneration. Brain 1989;112:1171–1192.

51. Graham NL, Bak TH, Patterson K, Hodges JR. Language function and dysfunction in corticobasal degeneration. Neurology 2003; 61:493–499.

52. Graham NL, Bak TH, Hodges JR. Corticobasal degeneration as a cognitive disorder. Mov Disord 2003;18(11):1224–1232.

53. Broussolle E, Bakchine S, Tommasi M, et al. Slowly progressive anarthria with late anterior opercular syndrome: a variant form of frontal cortical atrophy syndromes. J Neurol Sci 1996;144:444–458.

54. Soliveri P, Piacentini S, Carella F, et al. Progressive dysarthria: definition and clinical follow-up. Neurol Sci 2003;24:211–212.

55. Rosenbek JC. Mutism, neurogenic. In: Kent RD, ed. The MIT Encyclopedia of Communication Disorders. Cambridge, MA: MIT Press, 2004.

56. Yorkston KM, Miller RM, Strand EA. Management of Speech and Swallowing in Degenerative Diseases. 2nd ed. Austin, TX: PRO-ED, 2004.

57. Beukelman DR, Mirenda P. Augmentative and Alternative Communication: Management of Severe Communication Disorders in Children and Adults. 2nd ed. Baltimore: Paul H. Brookes, 1998.

58. Yorkston KM, Beukelman DR. Ataxic dysarthria: treatment sequences based on intelligibility and prosodic considerations. J Speech Hear Disord 1981;46(4):398–404.

59. Sapir S, Spielman J, Ramig LO, et al. Effects of intensive voice treatment (the Lee Silverman Voice Treatment [LSVT]) on ataxic dysarthria: a case study. Am J Speech Lang Pathol 2003;12(4):387–399.

60. Jones HN, Donovan NJ, Sapienza CM, et al. Expiratory muscle strength training in the treatment of mixed dysarthria in a patient with Lance Adams syndrome. J Med Speech Lang Pathol. In press.

61. Nagaya M, Kachi T, Yamada T, Sumi Y. Videofluorographic observations on swallowing in patients with dysphagia due to neurodegenerative diseases. Nagoya J Med Sci 2004;67(1–2):17–23.

62. Kronenbuerger M, Fromm C, Block F, et al. On-demand deep brain stimulation for essential tremor: a report on four cases. Mov Disord 2006;21(3):401–405.

63. Hamakawa S, Koda C, Umeno H, et al. Oropharyngeal dysphagia in a case of Huntington's disease. Auris Nasus Larynx 2004;31(2):171–176.

64. Kagel MC, Leopold NA. Dysphagia in Huntington's disease: a 16-year retrospective. Dysphagia 1992;7(2):106–114.

65. Kagel MC, Leopold NA. Dysphagia in Huntington's disease. Arch Neurol 1985;42(1):57–60.

66. Trejo A, Tarrats RM, Alonso ME, et al. Assessment of the nutrition status of patients with Huntington's disease. Nutrition 2004;20(2):192–196.

67. Oder W, Grimm G, Kollegger H, et al. Neurological and neuropsychiatric spectrum of Wilson's disease: a prospective study of 45 cases. J Neurol 1991;238(5):281–287.

68. Wang XH, Cheng F, Zhang F, et al. Living-related liver transplantation for Wilson's disease. Transpl Int 2005;18(6):651–656.

69. Stremmel W, Meyerrose K, Niederau C, et al. Wilson disease: clinical presentation, treatment, and survival. Ann Intern Med 1991;115(9):720–726.

70. Topaloglu H, Gucuyener K, Orkun C, Renda Y. Tremor of tongue and dysarthria as the sole manifestation of Wilson's disease. Clin Neurol Neurosurg 1990;92(3):295–296.

71. Liao KK, Wang SJ, Kwan SY, et al. Tongue dyskinesia as an early manifestation of Wilson disease. Brain Dev 1991;13(6):451–453.

72. Kumar TS, Moses PD. Isolated tongue involvement—an unusual presentation of Wilson's disease. J Postgrad Med 2005;51(4):337.

73. Pellecchia MT, Criscuolo C, Longo K, et al. Clinical presentation and treatment of Wilson's disease: a single-centre experience. Eur Neurol 2003;50(1):48–52.

74. Haggstrom G, Hirschowitz BI. Disordered esophageal motility in Wilson's disease. J Clin Gastroenterol 1980;2(3):273–275.

75. LaBlance GR, Rutherford DR. Respiratory dynamics and speech intelligibility in speakers with generalized dystonia. J Commun Disord 1991;24(2):141–156.

76. LaPointe LL, Case J, Duane D. Perceptual-acoustic speech and voice characteristics of subjects with spasmodic torticollis. In: Till J, Yorkston K, Beukelman D, eds. Motor Speech Disorders: Advances in Assessment and Treatment. Baltimore: Paul H. Brookes, 1994:40–45.

77. Golper LA, Nutt JG, Rau MT, Coleman RO. Focal cranial dystonia. J Speech Hear Disord 1983;48(2):128–134.

78. Tolosa E. Clinical Features of Meige's disease (idiopathic orofacial dystonia): a report of 17 cases. Arch Neurol 1981;38:147–151.

79. Edwards M, Schott G, Bhatia K. Episodic focal lingual dystonic spasms. Mov Disord 2003;18(7):836–837.

80. Baik JS, Park JH, Kim JY. Primary lingual dystonia induced by speaking. Mov Disord 2004;19(10):1251–1252.

81. Charles PD, Davis TL, Shannon KM, et al. Tongue protrusion dystonia: treatment with botulinum toxin. South Med J 1997;90(5):522–525.

82. Robertson-Hoffman DE, Mark MH, Sage JL. Isolated lingual/palatal dystonia. Mov Disord 1991;6(2):177–179.

83. Singer C, Papapetropoulos S. A comparison of jaw-closing and jaw-opening idiopathic oromandibular dystonia. Parkinsonism Relat Disord 2006;12(2):115–118.

84. Tan EK, Jankovic J. Bilateral hemifacial spasm: a report of five cases and a literature review. Mov Disord 1999;14(2):345–349.

85. Lagueny A, Burbaud P, LeMasson G, et al. Involvement of respiratory muscles in adult-onset dystonia: a clinical and electrophysiological study. Mov Disord 1995;10(6):708–713.

86. Lundy DS, Casiano RR, Lu FL, Xue JW. Abnormal soft palate posturing in patients with laryngeal movement disorders. J Voice 1996; 10(4):348–353.

87. Dworkin JP. Bite-block therapy for oromandibular dystonia. In: Cannito MP, Yorkston K, Beukelman D, eds. Neuromotor Speech Disorders: Nature, Assessment and Management. Baltimore: Paul H. Brookes, 1998.

88. Dworkin JP. Bite-block therapy for oromandibular dystonia. J Med Speech Lang Pathol 1996;4:47.

89. Brin MF, Fahn S, Moskowitz C, et al. Localized injections of botulinum toxin for the treatment of focal dystonia and hemifacial spasm. Mov Disord 1987;2:237–254.

90. Brin M, Blitzer A, Stewart C. Laryngeal dystonia (spasmodic dysphonia): observations of 901 patients and treatment with botulinum toxin. Adv Neurol 1998;78:237–252.

91. Tagliati M, Shils J, C. S, Alterman R. Deep brain stimulation for dystonia. Exp Rev Med Devices 2004;1(1):33–41.

92. Riski JE, Horner J, Jr. NB. Swallowing function in patients with spasmodic torticollis. Neurology 1990;40(9):1443–1445.

93. Cersosimo MG, Juri S, Suarez de Chandler S, et al. Swallowing disorders in patients with blepharospasm. Medicina 2005;65(2): 117–120.

94. Mascia MM, Valls-Sole J, Marti MJ, Sanz S. Chewing pattern in patients with Meige's syndrome. Mov Dis 2005;20(1):26–33.

95. Holzer SE, Ludlow CL. The swallowing side effects of botulinum toxin type A injection in spasmodic dysphonia. Laryngoscope 1996;106:86–92.

96. Horner J, Riski JE, Ovelmen-Levitt J, Nashold BSJ. Swallowing in torticollis before and after rhizotomy. Dysphagia 1992;7(3):117–125.

97. Feve A, Angelard B, Lacau St Guily J. Laryngeal tardive dyskinesia. J Neurol 1995;242(7):455–459.

98. Gerratt BR. Formant frequency fluctuation as an index of motor steadiness in the vocal tract. J Speech Hear Res 1983;26(2): 297–304.

99. Portnoy RA. Hyperkinetic dysarthria as an early indicator of impending tardive dyskinesia. J Speech Hear Disord 1979;44(2):214–219.

100. Frangos E, Christodoulides H. Clinical observations of the treatment of tardive dyskinesia with haloperidol. Acta Psychiatr Belg 1975; 75(1):19–32.
101. Kent RD, Kent JF, Rosenbek JC. Maximum performance tests of speech production. J Speech Hear Disord 1987;52:367–387.
102. Wertz RT, LaPointe LL, Rosenbek JC. Apraxia of Speech in Adults: The Disorder and Its Management. Orlando, FL: Grune & Stratton, 1984.

Appendix A
Grandfather Passage

You wish to know all about my grandfather. Well, he is nearly 93 years old, yet he still thinks as swiftly as ever. He dresses himself in an old black frock coat, usually with several buttons missing. A long beard clings to his chin, giving those who observe him a pronounced feeling of the utmost respect. Twice each day he plays skillfully and with zest upon a small organ. Except in the winter when the snow or ice prevents, he slowly takes a short walk in the open air each day. We have often urged him to walk more and smoke less, but he always answers, "Banana oil!" Grandfather likes to be modern in his language.

Source: From Duffy JR. Motor Speech Disorders. 2nd ed. Philadelphia: Elsevier, 2005, with permission.

Appendix B

Perceptual Features of Motor Speech Disorders

Flaccid dysarthria	Spastic dysarthria	Ataxic dysarthria	Hypokinetic dysarthria	Hyperkinetic dysarthria-chorea	Hyperkinetic dysarthria-dystonia	Apraxia of speech
Hypernasality*	Imprecise consonants*	Imprecise consonants	Monopitch	Imprecise consonants	Imprecise consonants	Consonant distortions
Imprecise consonants	Monopitch	Equal and excess stress*	Reduced stress	Prolonged intervals*	Distorted vowels*	Substitutions
Breathiness (continuous)*	Reduced stress	Irregular articulatory breakdowns*	Monoloudness	Variable rate*	Harsh vocal quality*	Distorted substitutions
Monopitch	Harshness	Distorted vowels*	Imprecise consonants	Monopitch	Irregular articulatory breakdowns*	Additions
Nasal emission*	Low pitch*	Harsh vocal quality	Inappropriate silences	Harsh vocal quality	Strained-strangled voice*	Distorted additions
Audible inspiration*	Slow rate*	Prolonged phonemes*	Short rushes of speech	Inappropriate silences*	Monopitch	Omissions
Harsh vocal quality	Strained-strangled voice*	Prolonged intervals	Harsh vocal quality	Distorted vowels	Monoloudness	Slow overall rate
Short phrases*	Short phrases	Monopitch	Breathy voice (continuous)	Excess loudness variations*	Inappropriate silences*	Syllable segregation
Monoloudness	Distorted vowels	Monoloudness	Low pitch	Prolonged phonemes*	Short phrases	Groping for articulatory postures
	Pitch breaks	Slow rate	Variable rate	Monoloudness	Prolonged intervals	Difficulty with initiation
		Excess loudness variations*	Increased rate in segments	Short phrases	Prolonged phonemes	
			Increase of rate overall*	Irregular articulatory breakdowns	Excess loudness variations*	
			Repeated phonemes*	Equal & excess stress	Reduced stress	

* Indicates features which may be more distinctive or severe than in other dysarthria types.

Source: Duffy JR. Motor Speech Disorders. 2nd ed. Philadelphia: Elsevier, 2005.

11

PHYSICAL AND OCCUPATIONAL THERAPY

Progressive physical disability that is not specifically addressed by current pharmacologic regimens is a common finding in patients with progressive movement disorders. Often, physical and occupational therapy are necessary and can be provided for management of these disorders. Both deficits of upper extremity function caused by apraxia or ataxia can result in defective movement. Deficits of walking and balance can also be targeted by physical and occupational therapy interventions.[1–3] This chapter discusses the role of physical and occupational therapists in the care and management of movement disorders. We will first discuss the role of physical and occupational therapists as part of the management team for Parkinson's disease, parkinsonism, and other movement disorders. We will subsequently discuss the specific issue of the falling patient. Finally, we will discuss emerging information on the impact of exercise on neurologic function.

ROLE OF PHYSICAL AND OCCUPATIONAL THERAPISTS IN MOVEMENT DISORDERS

Movement disorders are grouped together on the basis of similarity of clinical presentation. Many movement disorders represent progressive, multisystem neurodegenerative processes. A few important conceptual points are relevant to the clinical care of patients:

- Many movement disorders result in progressive disability over time.

  - Parkinsonism such as progressive supranuclear palsy (PSP), vascular parkinsonism (VP), multiple system atrophy (MSA), dementia with Lewy bodies (DLB), and corticobasal-ganglionic degeneration (CBDG) result in relatively rapid rates of decline.[4–7]

  - Idiopathic Parkinson's disease (PD) usually has a relatively slower rate of progression, but disabling medication unresponsive deficits will develop over time in a majority of patients.[8]

  - Hereditary choreas, ataxias, and dystonias similarly result in progressive decline at a variable rate which is dependant on the disease process.[9–11]

  - In all movement disorders, it must be considered that not only motor dysfunction, but cognitive and speech/swallowing deficits may develop over time.

- Disability in movement disorders occurs in defined domains.

  - Dexterity for performing activities of daily living (ADLs)

  - Gait and balance

  - Speech and swallowing function

  - Mood

  - Cognition

- Effective management strategies involve addressing these domains of disability.

  - Early in the course the focus can frequently be on correction of deficits

  - Later in the course of disease, the focus should shift to developing compensatory strategies.[1–3]

  - Lessening caregiver burden should be a defined management goal.[12]

Management of disability in movement disorders is not straightforward, and involves a multidisciplinary approach. Although this chapter focuses specifically on the roles of the physical therapist (PT) and the occupational therapist (OT) in the management

Table 11.1
The Management Team

Dexterity, gait, balance	Physical and occupational therapists
Swallow function, dysarthria, hypophonia	Speech pathology
Cognitive decline	Speech pathology, neuropsychology, pharmacist, occupational therapist
Mood disorders	Neurologist, primary care physician, psychiatrist

of movement disorders, these specialists should be thought of as part of a multidisciplinary team (Table 11.1).

The role of both the PT and OT in the treatment parkinsonism is to address motor dysfunction to increase functional independence. Dependence on others for ADLs is a primary reason patients seek treatment. This loss of function may contribute to a perceived decline in quality of life for patients.[13]

DIFFERENTIATING THE ROLES OF PHYSICAL AND OCCUPATIONAL THERAPISTS

Physical therapists and occupational therapists have separate areas of expertise (Figure 11.1), and a physician referring to one of these specialties should be familiar with the domains of expertise of each profession.[14–15]

Role of the PT

Postural instability and dysfunction of gait/balance are common symptoms in many movement disorders (Table 11.2). The goal of physical therapy is to teach patients exercises, strategies, and compensations that maintain or increase activity levels, decrease rigidity and bradykinesia, optimize gait, and improve balance and motor coordination.

When to Refer to a PT

Referral to a PT for early intervention should be considered when trying to manage the physical disability caused by PD. Referal will accomplish the following:

- Identify motor dysfunction as well as impairments that can be addressed through exercise and behavioral modification

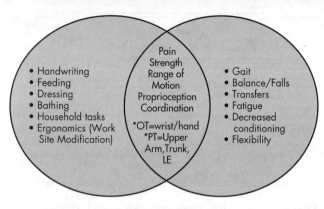

FIGURE 11.1
Differentiating the roles of the occupational therapist (left)
and the physical therapist (right).

	Table 11.2 PT Treatment Regimens
Deficit	Treatment
Deconditioning (cardio-vascular deconditioning, muscular weakness)	Strength training programs Endurance training
Rigidity	Range of motion and flexibility exercises
Postural instability	Balance training (Figure 11.2), postural adjustment exercises
Gait dysfunction	Adaptive stepping techniques • *Visual cues* (Figure 11.3; e.g., step over an object or caregiver's foot, inverted cane, using a laser pointer to create a dot on floor as a target) • *Auditory cues* (e.g., metronome, counting aloud, humming a tune) • *Internal cue*—for patients with mild disability who are able to concentrate on step-by-step activity rather than continuous gait. Patients can stop/pause to regroup/reset and start again with one good step.
Declining ability to perform activities of daily living	*Self-care:* exercises for improved bed mobility, transfers, dressing, grooming, bathing, eating, toileting *Home management:* shopping, chores, caregiving, yard work (collaborative care with occupational therapist)

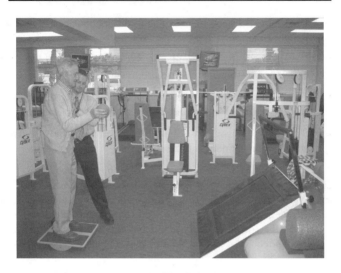

FIGURE 11.2

Example of balance training. Patient is standing on a "wobble board." The upper extremities are occupied with a task to mimic multitasking necessary in many ADLs.

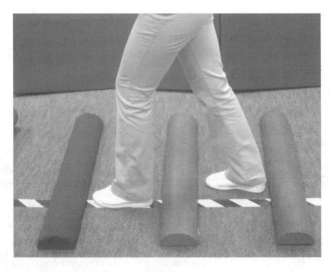

FIGURE 11.3

Example of stepping exercises. Patients with gait freezing develops a motor program of stepping by using visual cues.

- Determine the need for treatment and document changes in patient function

- Develop effective gait and balance strategies with greater ease before significant disease progression ensues

- Educate patients and families/caregivers about expected progression as well as the importance of the maintenance of exercises

- Slow development of disability due to poor cardiovascular conditioning or poor muscle strength

The role of the PT in current practice is to harness available circuitry to relearn skills that have been lost due to deficiencies in striatal function, whether this is due to dopamine deficiency or to other degenerative processes affecting the basal ganglia. The PT should be consulted early about patients who are falling or developing deficits of gait or balance.

Role of the OT

Deficits in dextrous movements, as well as progressive therapy-resistant deficits with gait and balance, are common in movement disorders (Table 11.3). The primary goal of the OT is to

Table 11.3
OT Treatment Regimens

Deficit	Treatment
Poor gait rhythm	Multisensory cueing, cognitive cueing strategies
Poor motor dexterity	Coordination drills
Fatigue	Energy conservation techniques
Declining ability to perform activities of daily living	*Self-care:* devices and techniques are provided to reduce dependence. Practice in a monitored setting with devices is necessary for devices to be incorporated in patient's activity routines. *Home management:* lightweight vacuum cleaners and dust mops, jar openers, long-handled scrub brushes, and other devices to may be considered to facilitate independence. Home assessments may be performed to evaluate for safety hazards such as throw rugs or for provision of adaptive devices such as handicap bars, shower seats, ramps, or other devices designed to improve function in the home.
Handwriting	Exercises to improve hand manipulation skills and independent finger movements (Figure 11.5).

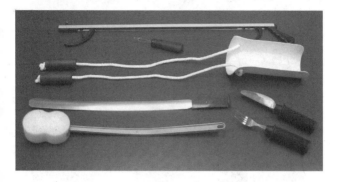

FIGURE 11.4
Example of adaptive devices.

assist in improving the quality of life throughout the disease process, by improving functional movement, and through proscription of adaptive devices to assist in maintaining independent functions.[16–20]

When to Refer to an OT

Early referral to an occupational therapist will address:

- Baseline evaluations of the degree of motor disorder, active functional movement, passive joint movement, dependence level in ADLs, speed of performance of self-care activities, handwriting skills, and ability to perform simultaneous and sequential tasks

- Instruction in accommodation principles that can be used throughout the progression of the disease

- Prevention of musculoskeletal deficits

- Instruction in grading of activities so function can be facilitated despite changing symptoms

- Early initiation of environmental adaptations

- Caregiver instruction in the disease process and the process of rehabilitation

- Patient and caregiver support

The OT uses a different set of strategies than the PT to improve function, and the best outcomes usually develop when the two disciplines work together.

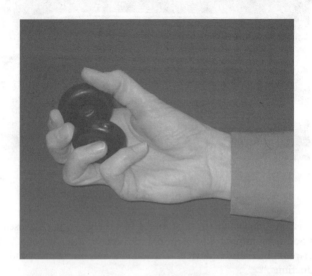

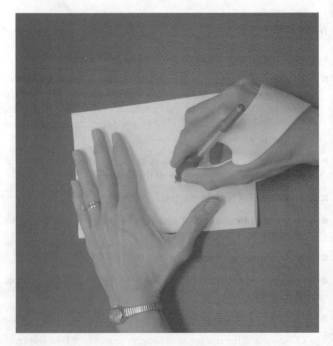

FIGURE 11.5
Example of writing exercises.

PHYSICAL AND OCCUPATIONAL THERAPY IN PARKINSON'S DISEASE

At initial diagnosis, physical and occupational therapy may or may not be required in PD. Functional disability related to symptoms may be manageable with medications. Over time, the strategy for management in PD shifts as the disease progresses. Early in the disease process, medication may correct deficits associated with bradykinesia, rigidity, and tremor. Strategies including physical and occupational therapists can be similarly weighted toward correction of deficits with practice oriented routines that focus on normalizing functional performance. Later, as functional performance continues to degrade, and particularly as medication-unresponsive deficits in gait and balance begin to develop, the focus needs to change to compensatory techniques such as altering techniques of sitting and standing, utilization of canes and walkers, and adaptive devices to assist with dressing, hygiene, and other ADLs such as opening cans and using utensils (Table 11.4).

In early Parkinson's disease (Hoehn and Yahr [H & Y] stages 1–2), corrective and compensatory strategies frequently maintain a high overall level of performance, and many patients with mild to moderate disease can continue to work in some capacity and perform ADLs without assistance. With the development of medication-unresponsive deficits in balance and gait (H & Y stage 3 and higher), compensatory strategies begin to have a more important role. In end stages of disease (H & Y stage 5), medication-unresponsive deficits become the primary disabling factors, and compensatory strategies to allow performance of ADLs may be required.

Table 11.4
Strategies for Modifying Disability in Parkinson's Disease

Hoehn and Yahr stage	Correction	Compensation
1	×	
2	×	×
3	×	×
4	×	×
5		×

PHYSICAL AND OCCUPATIONAL THERAPY IN PARKINSONISM AND IN OTHER MOVEMENT DISORDERS

The overall strategy for physical and occupational therapy in parkinsonism and other movement disorders is similar to the strategy in PD; however, initial functional disability upon diagnosis may be greater, medication responsiveness may be less, and the rate of decline in function can be steeper. Cases must be treated individually depending on specific needs.

THE FALLING PATIENT

Falls are a leading cause of morbidity and mortality in the elderly population and frequently contribute to the need for nursing home placement.[21] This is a particular issue in patients with movement disorders, which often result in deficits of gait and balance. For example, parkinsonism is a major risk factor for falls in surveys of the elderly.[22,23] Dystonia, chorea, and ataxia can similarly result in gait disturbances that predispose to falls. The following factors in movement disorders predispose to falling or increase the risk of falls in individuals with movement disorders:

- Older age

- Longer duration of disease

- Advanced disease stage

- Rigidity or dystonia of the lower limbs

- Freezing or festination

- Severe chorea or dyskinesia

- Ataxia

- Symptomatic orthostatic hypotension

- Other medical or neurologic conditions

- Local environmental factors

The clinician confronted with a patient who is falling should not assume that the cause of all falls is the same. Because falls or their basis may not be readily detected on physical examination, the clinician must take a careful history to determine the true frequency of falling and the potential causes and contributing

Table 11.5
Evaluating Falls in Movement Disorders

Source of fall	Associated disease processes	Evaluation
Postural instability	Parkinson's disease and parkinsonism	Retropulsion pull test: • Examiner stands behind the patient, usually in proximity to a wall, and gives a short tug backwards. Observation capacity to maintain balance by stepping backward is observed.
Freezing/start hesitation	Parkinson's disease and parkinsonism	Observe walking. Freezing can frequently be observed in enclosed spaces (e.g., a small exam room), during turns (turn hesitation), or when starting from a standing position (start hesitation).
Ataxia	Ataxias, Huntington's disease	Evaluate gait. Ataxic gait is wide based. Patients may weave. Tandem walking is impaired. Individuals are frequently not able to stand with feet together.
Medications	All	Medication history should be obtained. Drugs can contribute to falls, particularly psychoactive drugs, hypotensive medications, and alcohol.
Environmental	All	Environmental causes of falls may interact with any of the above sources of falling.

factors. Identification of the probable cause is important for developing an effective treatment plan. Table 11.5 discusses some common causes of falls in different movement disorders, and strategies for evaluating fall risk.

Managing Falls

Both festination and freezing and postural instability related to parkinsonism may respond to drug therapy early in the disease. However, ataxia does not usually respond to multimodality therapy, and patients with more advanced disease often fail to improve with pharmacologic therapy. Surgical therapy is only occasionally useful in patients with Parkinson's disease in which falls result from motor fluctuations, and surgical therapies such as deep brain stimulation rarely provide satisfactory results in Parkinson's disease when postural instability cannot be improved (even if only temporarily) with medical management.[24] Surgical intervention is ineffective for improving falls in parkinsonism or in ataxic disorders. In most patients who begin to fall because of postural instability, a few principal interventions are prudent:

- Physical therapy. Physical therapy may improve recognition of risk, and improve strength. Strategies for turning or providing a more stable base of support during activities may also be taught in this environment. Motor and sensory tricks may also be taught to improve freezing and festination.

- Occupational therapy. Assistive devices such as walkers may be useful.

- Home safety: Environmental factors leading to falls should be evaluated.

Table 11.6 details some specific strategies for managing falls.

Prevention is the best strategy for managing falls.[20] The underlying cause of falling should be determined and corrected if possible. In patients with postural instability or freezing, establishing the relationship between dopaminergic treatments and falls is crucial, as treatment alterations may improve falls. In all cases, an underlying medical or neurologic condition should be identified. Physical therapy can improve strength, cardiovascular fitness, and balance. Educating the patient and caregiver is also important. Environmental risk factors must be evaluated. However, not all risk factors are correctable, and even after optimal treatment many patients continue to experience falls. The use of a wheelchair may be the best solution for these patients.

CONCLUSION

A multidisciplinary management team is optimal for appropriately managing disability in movement disorders. Physical and occupational therapists can be important allies in a health-care team, and respecting the roles of these professionals is an important aspect of developing a good management team.

Table 11.6
Management of Falls in Movement Disorders

Source of fall	Management strategy
Postural instability	• Medical: Increased levodopa dosage may improve postural stability. • Surgical: If the source of falls is motor fluctuations in Parkinson's disease, then deep brain stimulation may be useful. • Physical therapy: Strategies for turning and for improving base of support may be taught. Strengthening can improve capacity to resist postural challenge in some patients. • Occupational therapy: Assistive devices are often useful.
Freezing/festination	• Medical: Increased levodopa dosage may improve postural stability. • Surgical: If freezing is related to motor fluctuations, then deep brain stimulation may be useful. • Physical therapy: Assisting patients to develop internal cueing such as counting or focusing on a single action (e.g., step over a crack in the floor) may be useful. Some individuals may use strategies such as stepping sideways or rocking the trunk back and forward to break a freezing episode; however care must be taken to avoid inducing a fall. • Occupational therapy: Visual stimuli may be presented on a cane or walker (such as a line produced by a laser) to improve stepping activity.
Ataxia	Both physical and occupational therapy may be useful to improve balance and adaption to disability.
Medications	Medications that may be contributing to falls should be adjusted or discontinued.
Environmental causes	Evaluation of the home environment is the pervue of occupational therapists. Specific interventions may be useful: • Footwear: Poorly fitting or nonsupportive footwear may result in falls. Nonskid shoes may augment freezing. An occupational therapist working in concert with a podiatrist may be able to suggest appropriate footwear. • Home visits may be useful to define safety harzards, such as: 1. Loose throw-rugs or torn carpeting 2. Covering slippery surfaces 3. Poor lighting conditions 4. Unsafe stairways

REFERENCES

1. Morris ME. Movement disorders in people with Parkinson disease: a model for physical therapy. Phys Ther 2000;80:578–597.

2. Umphred DA. (2001). Neurological rehabilitation. 4th ed. St. Louis: Mosby.

3. Trombly C, & Radomski M. Occupational therapy for physical dysfunction. 5th ed. Philadelphia: Lippincott Williams & Wilkins, 2002.

4. Nath U. Clinical features and natural history of progressive supranuclear palsy: a clinical cohort study.*Neurology* 2003;60(6):910–916.

5. Wenning GK . Multiple system atrophy. *Lancet Neurol* 2004; 3(2): 93–103

6. Christine CW. Clinical differentiation of parkinsonian syndromes: prognostic and therapeutic relevance. *Am J Med* 2004; 117(6): 412–9.

7. Thanvi B, Lo N, & Robinson T. Vascular parkinsonism—an important cause of parkinsonism in older people. Age Ageing. 2005;34(2): 114–119.

8. Hauser RA. Current treatment challenges and emerging therapies in Parkinson's disease. Neurol Clin 2004; 22(3):

9. Anderson KE . Huntington's disease and related disorders. *Psychiatr Clin North Am* 2005;28(1):275–290.

10. Mariotti C. An overview of the patient with ataxia. J Neurol 2005; 252(5):511–588.

11. Defazio G. Epidemiology of primary dystonia. *Lancet Neurol* 2004; 3(11):673–678.

12. Smallegan M. How families decide on nursing home admission. Geriatr Consult 1983;1:21–24.

13. Karlson K, Larson J, Tandberg E, & Maeland J. Influences of clinical and demographic variables in quality of life in patients with Parkinson's disease. J Neurol Neuropsychiatry Psychiatry 66: 431–435, 1999.

14. Guide to Physical Therapist Practice. 2nd ed.Alexandria, VA: American Physical Therapy Association, 2003.

15. Trombly C, & Radomski M. Occupational Therapy for Physical Dysfunction. 5th ed. Philadelphia: Lippincott Williams & Wilkins, 2002.

16. Byl NN, & Melnick ME. The neural consequences of repetition: Clinical implications of a learning hypothesis. J Hand Ther 1997; 10:160–172.

17. Cornhill M. In-hand manipulation: The association to writing skills. Am J Occup Ther 1996;50:732–739.

18. Gauthier L, Dalziel S, & Gauthier S. The benefits of group occupational therapy for patients with Parkinson's disease. Am J Occupl Ther 1987;41(6):360–365.

19. Murphy S, & Tickle-Degnen L. The effectiveness of occupational therapy-related treatments for persons with Parkinson's disease: A meta-analytic review. Am J Occup Ther 2001;55(4):385–392.

20. Pedretti LW. Occupational Therapy Practice Skills for Physical Dysfunction. 4th ed. St. Louis: Mosby, 1996.

21. Smallegan M. How families decide on nursing home admission. Geriatr Consult 1983;1:21–24.

22. Tinetti ME, Speechley M, & Ginter SF. Risk factors for falls among elderly persons living in the community. N Engl J Med 1988;319: 1701–1707.
23. Nevitt MC, Cummings SR, Kidd S, & Black D. Risk factors for recurrent nonsyncopal falls. A prospective study. JAMA 1989;261: 2663–2668
24. Olanow CW, Watts RL, & Koller WC. An algorithm (decision tree) for the management of Parkinson's disease: Treatment guidelines. Neurology 2001;56(11): S1–S88.

12

NUTRITIONAL CONSIDERATIONS

Good nutrition is essential to maintaining well-being in individuals with neurologic disease. There are several reasons why nutrition is important in movement disorders:

■ Nutrition may impact mobility, cognition, and swallowing function. Movement disorders by definition result in changes in mobility, and may lead to a decreased capacity to perform activities of daily living such as cooking and shopping.

■ Cognitive dysfunction may impact the capacity to plan healthy meals.

■ Parkinson's disease, the parkinsonisms, and many causes of chorea and ataxia can be associated with dysphagia.

■ Poor nutrition in movement disorders may contribute to weight loss. Conversely, decreased levels of activity may lead to a sedentary lifestyle and obesity, exacerbating the underlying neurologic disability.

■ Finally, individuals with movement disorders frequently actively pursue both traditional and nontraditional treatment regimens, vitamin therapies, and herbal remedies which are frequently proposed for management of many symptoms.

Patients will often discuss nutrition with their primary neurologist or primary-care physician. All of the above reasons suggest that physicians caring for individuals with movement disorders have a familiarity with appropriate nutritional strategies for patients with movement disorders. This chapter is structured to discuss nutritional issues with respect to the various movement disorders (Parkinson's disease, the parkinsonisms, Huntington's disease, choreiform disorders, dystonia, and ataxia), and will be followed by sections discussing management of the malnourished patient and nutritional supplements.

THE MALNOURISHED PATIENT

Unintended Weight Loss in Movement Disorders

Unintended weight loss is a decrease in body weight that is not voluntary. Weight loss can occur with decreased food intake, increased metabolism, or both. Individuals with movement disorders should be periodically weighed as part of a routine neurologic evaluation. Significant weight loss (<10% of body weight) that is unintended should prompt a discussion of potential causes. The parkinsonisms, choreiform disorders, essential tremor, and ataxic disorders can all similarly be associated with weight loss. Weight loss in movement disorders may not only be due to decreased intake, but may also be related to changes in energy demands (in some cases, individuals with severe tremor, dyskinesias, or chorea may also have associated weight loss).[1-2] Unintentional weight loss may have common causes across movement disorders (Figure 12.1).

■ *Decreased ability to swallow.* Patients who have trouble swallowing eat more slowly, they are satiated (satisfied) more easily, and eat less.

■ *Decreased appetite.* Apathy, anxiety, or depression frequently accompany movement disorders such as Huntington's disease and Parkinson's disease, and may result in decreased interest in food or food preparation. Drugs such as Sinemet (carbidopa/levodopa) may cause nausea or decreased appetite. Changes in sensation, such as a decreased sense of smell (a common finding in Parkinson's disease) may result in decreased taste and craving for food.

■ *Poor oral hygiene.* Motor deficits with difficulties performing activities of daily living (ADLs) such as attending to hygiene needs may contribute to poor dentition, impacting nutrition.

■ *Elevated energy needs.* Patients who have frequent, moderate to marked tremors, dyskinesia, or rigidity may burn calories faster.

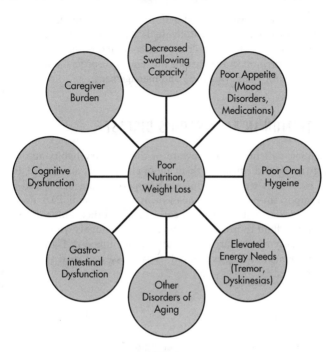

FIGURE 12.1

Factors leading to poor nutrition in movement disorders.

- *Psychosocial factors.* Individuals with advancing disease may progressively burden caregivers, sometimes overwhelming the capacity of caregivers to provide adequate care.

- *Gastrointestinal dysfunction.* In many disorders, such as Parkinson's disease and multiple systems atrophy, autonomic dysfunction can impact gut function, causing reflux, constipation, and other problems.

- *Executive dysfunction.* Cognitive dysfunction, particularly difficulties with planning and coordinating of complex activities, can impact the capacity to plan and cook meals in individuals with limited support networks.

- *Other disorders of aging.* Although weight loss may be a unique feature of many movement disorders, unplanned weight loss may also be a sign of other medical illnesses such as malignancy, gastrointestinal defects, chronic infections, and endocrinologic defects.

Nutritional intervention and assessment are an important component of overall care in individuals with movement disorders. The purpose of this chapter is to discuss factors that may result in poor nutrition in the various movement disorders and discuss strategies for their evaluation and management.

NUTRITION IN PARKINSON'S DISEASE

Helping patients become aware of their dietary habits and energy needs and educating them about elements of a balanced diet as well as in techniques for altering poor eating habits can be an important part of the management of nutrition in Parkinson's disease (PD). Patients should eat a balanced diet with sufficient fiber and fluid to prevent constipation. Individuals with PD may have many of the barriers to nutrition identified in Figure 12.1. Management strategies tailored to each assessed need should be formulated.

Dysphagia

Increased oral transit time is a common finding in PD. Management includes:

- Referral for speech therapy for any patient who complains of choking or problems with swallowing. Alterations in swallowing technique may help with function.

- Changes in food consistency (soft diet) for some patients.

Decreased Appetite

Individuals with weight loss should specifically be asked about appetite. Dopaminergic therapy can change appetite. Levodopa, for example, commonly decreases appetite, and may cause nausea. Dopamine agonists, on the other hand, may increase appetite. Mood may impact appetite. Management may include:

- Taking levodopa with a meal. Since there is an interaction between levodopa and dietary protein (see section on Other Considerations below), changing timing of levodopa dosing should be individualized.

- Evaluation/treatment of anxiety or depression.

Elevated Energy Needs

Treatment should be tailored to the patient.

- Mild dyskinesias are frequently necessary to maintain good motor function in levodopa-sensitive patients in the later stages of PD, and are not necessarily a reason to alter medical therapy. Increased dietary caloric intake is an appropriate management strategy.

- In patients with severe dyskinesias sufficient to alter energy requirements, changes in medication including lower overall levodopa dosage may help mitigate symptoms.

- Severe tremor can increase energy requirements, and can be a significant nuisance to quality of life. Increasing levodopa dosage or adding an agonist or an anticholinergic may be helpful.

- If medication alterations are not helpful for severe tremor or dyskinesia, deep brain stimulation may be considered in select patients.

Autonomic Dysfunction

Autonomic dysfunction is a common complication of PD. Although overshadowed by motor dysfunction in many patients, a large number of patients with PD experience significant dysautonomias including constipation, urinary problems, impotence, orthostasis, impaired thermoregulation, and sensory disturbances. GI manifestations may in particular impact nutrition.

- *Gastroesophageal reflux.* Poor transit through the stomach can lead to reflux of acid into the esophagus. Gastroesophageal reflux is treatable and should not be overlooked as a cause of nausea in PD. If reflux is present, use of small meals and avoidance of trigger foods such caffeine, citrus, tomatoes, and alcohol should be sought as a first-line treatment. Numerous small meals and snacks, nutrient dense and moderate in fat and fiber, may be helpful. The day's final meal should be consumed at least 4 hours before bedtime, so that the stomach is empty before lying down.

- *Constipation.* There is evidence that the neurodegenerative process may impact constipation. Lewy body deposition has been discovered in the myenteric plexus of patients with PD.[3]

Slowed stool transit time may result in constipation, with changes in appetite related to a feeling of fullness and intestinal discomfort. Dietary changes form the keystone of good management for PD. Specific recommendations for management include:

- Drink at least eight glasses of water a day.

- Eat high-fiber raw vegetables in at least two meals per day.

- Oat bran and other high-fiber additives may be helpful.

- Avoid baked goods and bananas.

- Avoid chronic laxative use, including senna, and cascara sagrada, as these may damage the colon and increase risk for cancer.

- Increase physical activity (walking and swimming are good).

- *Apomorphine in PD constipation.* Some practitioners have suggested that a paradoxical contraction of the pelvic floor musculature consistent with a pelvic floor dystonia may occur in some patients, leading to poor colonic emptying. In one study, defecatory function was improved in eight patients with PD after administration of apomorphine.[4]

- *Xerostomia (dry mouth).* Some anticholinergic medications, such as artane or medications used for bladder dysfunction, can cause dry mouth. Long-term effects of dry mouth include increased dental caries and gingivitis, and can be a significant problem in individuals who already have deficits in performing ADLs including oral hygiene. Stopping the offending medication if possible is usually the only effective therapy.

- *Cognitive and psychosocial factors.* Caregivers of individuals with PD face increasing caregiver burden with time, especially spouses, and particularly in later stages of disease when there exists a higher rate of depression for caregivers.[5] Caregivers may themselves be ill or older. Increasing problems with ADLs may result in decreased overall hygiene, including decreased oral hygiene (which may impact capacity to eat). Evidence of malnutrition in a PD patient should prompt a full psychosocial evaluation, including:

  - Home physical therapy and occupational therapy evaluation to evaluate living mileau

  - Social work interaction to evaluate caregiver resources

- ■ Dental evaluation if there is evidence of dental disease

- ■ Neuropsychologic evaluation to gauge the presence of significant dementia interfering with function

■ *Other disorders.* Individuals with PD are subject to other disorders of aging, and abrupt changes in weight or appetite should prompt consideration of other potential medical causes, including malignancy or endocrinologic abnormalities.

Other Nutritional Considerations in PD

Medical management in PD has significant nutritional ramifications. Dopaminergic medications in some patients may cause nausea and vomiting. In other cases, medications may cause other side effects that impact nutrition. Conversely, protein intake may interfere with medication absorption. The impact of medical therapy on overall nutritional status should be attended to. Specific issues include:

■ *Levodopa-related nausea and vomiting.* Initiation of levodopa may cause nausea and vomiting. Management strategies to mitigate levodopa-induced nausea include:

- ■ When starting patients on levodopa, start at an initial dose of 1/2 tablet tid to decrease chance of nausea.

- ■ Initially, patients may need to take levodopa with food.

- ■ Ginger tea and chewing crystallized ginger may help in some patients.

- ■ Extra carbidopa (25- to 50-mg dose, taken with levodopa) may help mitigate peripheral effects of levodopa, including nausea (also a medication called domperidone may help nausea).

■ *Levodopa-protein interaction.* Large neutral amino acids compete with levodopa uptake both from the gut and across the blood-brain barrier. Interactions between protein and levodopa usually become evident in patients in later stages of PD. Management strategies include:

- ■ Using the immediate-release formulation of levodopa, taken 30 minutes before meals.

- ■ Protein restriction during the day has been recommended by some practitioners.[6] This strategy works as a short-term solution, but may not be as effective as a long-term solution.[3]

- ■ Carbidopa (Lodosyn) and domperidone can combat nausea and vomiting in extreme cases.

- ■ Proclorperazine (Compazine) and metoclopramide (Reglan) are to be avoided, as they block dopamine receptors and increase parkinsonian symptoms.

- ■ In selected patients in whom motor fluctuations cannot be well controlled, deep brain stimulation surgery is a consideration.

■ *Unplanned weight gain due to dopaminergic drugs.* Unplanned weight gain can occur related to dopamine agonists such as pramipexole (Mirapex) or ropinirole (Requip). Both may cause increased caloric intake, or they may increase fluid retention. Compulsive eating may also occur. Amantadine may also increase fluid retention. Management may include:

- ■ Increased physical activity.

- ■ Decreased salt intake may help in some cases.

- ■ Discontinuation or alteration of the dose of the offending medication may be necessary.

- ■ Obsessive behaviors related to dopamine agonists are idiosyncratic and do not appear to be strictly dose related. Typically, these problems are not treatable except by stopping the offending medication. Observation of obsessive eating should prompt questions about other obsessive behaviors, such as gambling or sexual obsessions.

- ■ DBS may also result in weight gain for unclear reasons.

NUTRITION IN THE PARKINSONISMS

Management of nutrition in the parkinsonisms is similar to management in PD. In many cases, dysphagia is a larger and more significant cause of poor nutrition. Specific issues relevant to individual disorders are discussed below.

Multiple System Atrophy

Patients with multiple system atrophy (MSA) have unique pharmacologic challenges related nutrition. In many cases, autonomic instability with orthostasis is a significant cause of disability.

Many patients are levodopa responsive, but levodopa may have significant side effects, impacting blood pressure. Blood pressure fluctuations may also occur related to digestion of meals. Dysphagia may also impact nutrition. Issues related to nutrition in MSA may include:

- *Dysphagia.* Individuals with MSA may develop choking or difficulties swallowing, and aspiration. Management includes:

  - Speech pathologists should be part of the management team, and should be consulted early.

  - As dysphagia can become significant later in the disease process, it is reasonable to ascertain early patient wishes with respect to feeding tubes and other supportive nutritional devices.

- *Gastrointestinal dysfunction.* Autonomic dysfunction impacting the GI tract is similar to that found in idiopathic PD, but frequently more severe. Management is similar to management in PD.

- *Postprandial hypotension.* This complication commonly occurs 30 to 90 minutes after eating a meal. Hypotension can be significant, and result in syncope and falls. Management includes:

  - Limiting meal size, with more frequent meals.

  - Midodrine 5–10 mg may be taken prior to meals to increase adrenergic tone after meals. **Midodrine should not be given within 4 hours of sleep.**

  - Limit levodopa dose. Impact of levodopa on motor function must be balanced against impact on blood pressure.

- *Cognitive dysfunction.* Executive dysfunction can become a significant source of disability and caregiver strain later in the disease process, and should be managed in a multidisciplinary fashion.

- *Increased energy requirements.* Later in the disease process, patients are less mobile, prone to develop pressure sores, and may develop a catabolic metabolism as the capacity to take food by mouth declines. Management can be challenging and strategy should be based on the wishes of the family and patient.

Progressive Supranuclear Palsy

Patients with progressive supranuclear palsy (PSP) are rarely very levodopa responsive, and medications interact less with nutrition than in PD or MSA. Dysphagia and executive dysfunction are significant sources of disability. Management includes:

- *Dysphagia.* Aspiration is a common cause of mortality in PSP. A speech pathologist should be consulted early. End of life issues should be discussed early, before cognitive dysfunction prevents the capacity to make decisions.

- *Executive dysfunction.* Executive dysfunction is a significant cause of disability in PSP. Individuals develop significant cognitive changes relatively early in the course of the disease, increasing caregiver burden.

- *Apraxia.* Individuals with PSP and parkinsonism associated with dementia may develop progressive bradykinesia and apraxia of limb movements. This type of apraxia may impact eating behavior. The supranuclear gaze palsy together with neck rigidity frequently interferes in later stages of the disease with looking down at the plate. Consequently, individuals with PSP develop progressive problems with self-feeding.

- *Increased energy requirements.* Later in the disease process, patients are less mobile, prone to develop pressure sores, and may develop a catabolic metabolism as the capacity to take food by mouth declines. Management of PSP, MSA, and parkinsonism in the end stages is challenging and should be based on the wishes of the family and patient.

Other Parkinsonisms

Corticobasal-ganglionic degeneration (CBGD) and other causes of parkinsonism including vascular parkinsonism typically require similar management strategies to those delineated for PD, MSA, and PSP.

NUTRITION IN CHOREIFORM DISORDERS

Choreiform disorders comprise a vast landscape of disease processes (see Chapter 11). Although the causes of these disorders vary, phenomenologically, the disorders share similar issues with respect to nutrition.

- *Increased energy requirements.* Increased energy demands due to chorea may require increased caloric intake. In Huntington's disease, increased chorea is associated with weight loss.[1] Nutritional plans should be made in order to allow for the increased energy demands of individuals who have significant chorea.

- *Dysphagia.* Dysphagia is a common complaint in nearly all choreiform disorders (with the exception of tardive dyskinesia). The speech pathologist is an important part of the management team for all of these disorders.

- *Chorea.* Chorea may occasionally interfere with self-feeding.

- *Cognitive and mood changes.* These are common in all of these disorders, and can impact the caregiver burden as well as the capacity to develop appropriate nutritional plans.

NUTRITION IN THE ATAXIC PATIENT

Genetic causes of ataxia overlap in many cases with genetic causes of chorea (see Chapter 11). Ataxia brings specific challenges to nutrition, many of which have been discussed in previous sections with respect to other movement disorders.

- *Dysphagia.* This is a common finding and warrants referral for swallowing evaluation. As in many of the movement disorders, the speech pathologist is an integral part of the team.

- *Ataxia.* Ataxia can significantly interfere with feeding. In some patients, a cerebellar or rubral tremor may prevent the patient from being able to bring food to the mouth. Occupational therapy may be able to assist with weighted utensils or other devices that allow feeding.

NUTRITIONAL DERANGEMENTS AS A CAUSE OF MOVEMENT DISORDERS

Although rare, a limited number of movement disorders are caused by aberrant nutritional absorption. Wilson's disease is caused by aberrant copper metabolism. Vitamin E deficiency can cause ataxia. Disorders of iron storage can cause chorea and ataxia. Specific nutritional requirements may be required for some diseases based on the diagnosis.

SWALLOWING DYSFUNCTION IN MOVEMENT DISORDERS

It is appropriate to close our discussion of barriers to nutrition in movement disorders by briefly discussing swallowing dysfunction. Swallowing dysfunction is a common feature of many movement disorders.[7] Oropharyngeal dysphagia (abnormal swallowing) may result in many complications, including dehydration, malnutrition, bronchospasm, and airway obstruction, as well as aspiration pneumonia and chronic chest infection. Secondary consequences of poor swallowing function may include increased caregiver strain, social isolation, and depression,[8] and therefore swallowing dysfunction may become a substantial component of disability. Evidence of aspiration, such as coughing or choking during meals, should be elicited during routine history. Management of dysphagia in movement disorders is covered elsewhere in this textbook; however, prompt referral to a speech pathologist is mandatory in any patients with complaints of swallowing dysfunction.

EVIDENCE ON NUTRITIONAL SUPPLEMENTS

A large body of literature has been developed in support of the hypothesis that oxidative stress is a contributing factor in the pathophysiology of many neurodegenerative diseases.[8,9] This literature led to the hypothesis that nutritional supplements that alter "scavengers" or the generation of free radicals might alter the progression of neurodegenerative disease. Multiple nutritional supplements have been proposed. Well-designed studies are lacking for any but a few nutritional supplements; owing in part to the large number of contenders in the field and to a lack of consensus on appropriate trial design. No nutritional agent has to date been shown to have the capacity to alter the course of any neurodegenerative disease.[10] As nutrition is a subject that is frequently brought up by patients, it is appropriate for clinicians to have some familiarity with research in this area. A discussion of nutritional supplements that have been formally evaluated in well-designed clinical studies follows.

■   Vitamins C and E both have antioxidant properties, which has prompted some practitioners to tout these vitamins as potential neuroprotective agents. Moreover, vitamin C can elevate levodopa levels, theoretically leading to potential symptomatic effects.[11] A nonrandomized, unblinded study suggested that combining vitamins E and C might slow the rate of progression in patients with early PD[12]; however, a randomized, blinded study of high-dose vitamin E alone using initiation of levodopa as a surrogate marker did not show any difference between the vitamin E and a placebo group.[13] A trial of vitamin E in Huntington's disease showed no improvement in the primary outcome variables (neuropsychologic change).[14] A fairly large literature exists on vitamins E and C in the prevention or treatment of Alzheimer's dementia; however, randomized, well-controlled studies are lacking, and there is currently no clear evidence from the dementia literature that either vitamin alone or in combination affects neurologic function in the dementias.[15] There is therefore no evidence to recommend vitamin E treatment to patients with movement disorders. There is currently insufficient evidence to evaluate if vitamin C might have disease-modifying effects.

- Mitochondrial dysfunction has been demonstrated in idiopathic PD. Coenzyme Q is an important intermediary in the respiratory chain. A single randomized, blinded safety and efficacy study of coenzyme Q showed a positive trend ($P = .09$) in individuals at the higher 1200-mg dose of coenzyme Q, with less disability as shown by decreased change in the Unified Parkinson Disease Rating Scale (UPDRS) from baseline.[16] An initial study of coenzyme Q in Huntington's disease, however, showed no change in rate of decline.[17] Further studies in specific disease populations will need to be performed in order to evaluate if coenzyme Q alters neurodegeneration.

- Recent studies have shown creatine to be safe in Huntington's disease and reduce some laboratory biomarkers proposed to reflect progressive neuronal damage.[18,19] Doses of 8 g per day were well tolerated. Creatine has also been studied in a randomized, double-blind fashion in a "futility trial" designed to evaluate if further studies of the supplement are warranted in PD.[20] No definitive evidence of alteration of clinical function has been demonstrated, but further studies of creatine in both disorders are ongoing based on preliminary work. Further studies will be needed to evaluate if creatine is an effective treatment to slow disease progression in either disorder.

CONCLUSION

Individuals with movement disorders often have barriers to appropriate nutrition. Decreased ability to swallow, poor appetite, elevated energy needs, and psychosocial and cognitive factors may all impact ability to maintain proper nutrition. Clinical attention to nutrition in these disorders is useful to prevent further disability. Including a speech pathologist and a nutritionist on the multidisciplinary team caring for individuals with these neurodegenerative diseases will improve outcomes.

REFERENCES

1. Mahant N, McCusker EA, Byth K, et al. Huntington's disease: clinical correlates of disability and progression. Neurology 2003;61(8): 1085–1892.

2. Uc EY, Struck LK, Rodnitzky RL, et al. Predictors of weight loss in Parkinson's disease. Mov Disord 2006;21(7):930–936.

3. Olanow CW, Watts RL, Koller WC. An algorithm (decision tree) for the management of Parkinson's disease (2001): treatment guidelines. Neurology 2001;56(11):S1–S88.

4. Edwards LL, Quigley EM, Harrned RK, et al. Defecatory function in Parkinson's disease: response to apomorphine. Ann Neurol 1993; 33(5):490–493.

5. Carter JH, Stewart BJ, Archbold PG, et al. Living with a person who has Parkinson's disease: the spouse's perspective by stage of disease. Mov Disord 1998;13(1):20–28.

6. Pincus JH. Influence of dietary protein on motor fluctuations in Parkinson's disease. Arch Neurol 1987;44(3):270–272.

7. Hammond CA, Goldstein LB. Cough and aspiration of food and liquids due to oral-pharyngeal dysphagia. ACCP Evidence-Based Clinical Practice Guidelines. Chest 2006;129(1 Suppl):186S–196S.

8. Olenow CW. A radical hypothesis for neurodegeneration. Trends Neurosci 1993;16:439–444.

9. Simonian NA, Coyle JT. Oxidative stress in neurodegenerative disease. Ann Rev Pharmacol Toxicol 1996;36:53–106.

10. Suchowersky O, Gronseth G, Perimutter J, et al. Practice parameter: Neuroprotective strategies and alternative therapies for Parkinson disease (an evidence-based review). Neurology 2006;66:976–982.

11. Ferry P, Johnson M, Wallis P. Use of complementary therapies and non-prescribed medication in patients with Parkinson's disease. Postgrad Med J 2002; 78:612–614.

12. Fahn S. A pilot trial of high-dose alpha-tocopherol and ascorbate in early Parkinson's disease. Ann Neurol 1992;32(Suppl):S128–S132.

13. The Parkinson Study Group. Effects of tocopherol and deprenyl on the progression of disability in early Parkinson's disease. N Engl J Med 1993; 328:176–183.

14. Peyser CE, Folstein M, Chase GA, et al. Trial of d-alpha-tocopherol in Huntington's disease. Am J Psychiatry 1995;152(12):1771–1775.

15. Boothby LA, Doering PL. Vitamin C and vitamin E for Alzheimer's disease. Ann Pharmacother 2005;39(12):2073–2080. Epub Oct 14, 2005. Review.

16. Shults CW, Oakes D, Kieburtz K, et al. Effects of coenzyme Q10 in early Parkinson's disease: evidence of slowing of functional decline. Arch Neurol 2002;8:271–276.

17. Huntington Study Group. A randomized, placebo-controlled trial of coenzyme Q10 and remacemide in Huntington's disease. Neurology 2001;57(3):397–404.

18. Hersch SM, Gevorkian S, Marder K, et al. Creatine in Huntington disease is safe, tolerable, bioavailable in brain and reduces serum 8OH2'dG. Neurology 2006;66(2):250–252.

19. Bender A, Auer DP, Merl T, et al. Creatine supplementation lowers brain glutamate levels in Huntington's disease. J Neurol 2005; 252(1):36–41.

20. NINDS NET-PD Investigators. A randomized, double-blind, futility clinical trial of creatine and minocycline in early Parkinson disease. Neurology 2006;66(5):664–71. Epub Feb 15, 2006.

INDEX

Note: Boldface numbers indicate illustrations; *t* indicates a table.